ECG Holter

Jan Adamec · Richard Adamec

ECG Holter

Guide to Electrocardiographic Interpretation

Foreword I by Prof. Lukas Kappenberger
Foreword II by Prof. Philippe Coumel

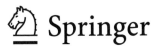 Springer

Jan Adamec
Cardiology Centre
University Hospital Geneva and
  Clinique La Prairie
Montreux, Vaud, Switzerland

Richard Adamec
Geneva, Switzerland

ISBN: 978-0-387-78186-0   e-ISBN: 978-0-387-78187-7
DOI: 10.1007/978-0-387-78187-7

Library of Congress Control Number: 2008920624

To Maureen and Kilian

Foreword I

For centuries the analysis of the heart rhythm has belonged to the foundations of medical art. We know that doctors in ancient Tibet used the interpretation of the heart rate to draw prognostic conclusions—somehow a modern rationale—that deserves further attention.

The rapid advancement of science is providing more and more information about the details, but the subatomic resolution of structures hides the risk and the complex procedures are fragmented into static impressions. The same has happened to the ECG. The revolutionary development, acknowledged by the Nobel Prize for Einthoven, led from the analysis of the dynamic heart rate to the static analysis of the heartstream curve. It is only with the ECG Holter recording over longer periods that the cardiologists rediscovered the old dynamic. With the continuous recording of the heart rate and its periodicity, it became accessible to a new dimension, a dimension that requires technically well-defined foundations for accurate data collection, detailed knowledge of the electrocardiologic particularities of arrhythmia, and medical knowledge for the translation of the results into a diagnostic synthesis.

With the ECG Holter the issue is no longer just to detect an arrhythmia, but also to determine dynamic circumstance in which the critical event occurred. In fact, we investigate the trigger, the event, and the context, and we have to integrate all of that information within the clinical picture, from the pathology right through to the symptom—indeed a multi-dimensional task.

In this volume the practice of 24-hr ECG recording is elucidated in detail, including discussion of the technical bases of the recording and the potential artefacts. There is a risk of wrong conclusions because of an excess of data. Avoiding errors in the data analysis is impossible without the assistance of IT (information technology), which means that we have to rely on an automatic interpretation, at least in terms of a preliminary triage.

Rightly, great interest is attributed to the formal analysis of the ECG, but one should be cautious about overemphasising the findings. It has been wrongly concluded for too long that trivial arrhythmias, as, for example, isolated ventricular premature beats, may trigger complex arrhythmias. Wrongly, it has been assumed that pharmaceutical suppression can inhibit ventricular tachycardias and fibrillation, and this false association has dominated the rhythmology and the therapy of tachycardias for several decades. Nowadays, though, there is a concensus that the trigger of dangerous arrhythmias cannot be identified without knowing the specific substrate. Therefore, these authors have to be acknowledged for not having correlated the exact electrocardiographic analysis with the therapeutic need for treatment.

The 24-hr ECG is designed to relate symptoms to electrocardiographic signs. Typically though, symptoms only rarely correlate with arrhythmias. This finding may reassure an anxious patient and help to forestall further expensive investigation. On the other hand, indications for heart disorders may be detected that justify further complementary investigations. In this context the recording take on a prognostic value—and hereby we return to Tibetan medicine.

The efficiency of therapeutic intervention, such as the treatment of atrial fibrillation or the implantation of pacemakers or defibrillators, can be surveyed. The present Holter guide focuses on the exact conventional ECG analysis and leaves the way open to new analytical methods such as frequency variability and QT-variation.

Only through clear-cut clinical demand and precise data analysis will the ECG Holter contribute to the diagnosis and therapy instituted. Otherwise, the technique will dominate the diagnostic, which we would like to avoid. Rightly, Jan and Richard Adamec remind us to be cautious regarding these risks, and in so doing they underscore their extensive practical and clinical experience in exposing the highly complex, but overall transparent, method of N. J. Holter.

Professor of Cardiology   Lukas Kappenberger
Lausanne University
Former President European Heart Rhythm Association

Foreword II

Norman Holter introduced a new time dimension in electrocardiography, but, curiously, it took a long time for the cardiologic community to fully appreciate the value of his approach.

A quarter of a century of clinical use has passed during which there has been a technological evolution from the electronic age to the computer era, but the technique of dynamic electrocardiography is still known by the inventor's name and we prescribe a "Holter" or we read one. We might ask ourselves why we do not prescribe an "Einthoven," for the latter has the advantage of having received a Nobel Prize for his invention more than a century ago. Concerning the Holter, all the repercussions of its innovation are not yet known, but let us think about what new developments we can expect. It is not one single channel anymore, but the entirety of the surface-numerised ECG which is within reach for the whole circadian period.

This manual by Richard and Jan Adamec reflects the long-term experience of the former and we can imagine that one day it will be extended by the latter with applications which have not yet been seen in clinical practice. Everything that concerns the clinical cardiologist in the "real world" figures in these pages and, more than that, the volume also touches on the philosophy with which one should approach Holter recordings. The reading by a technician is used largely for practical reasons, but there is no more evidence in favour of giving a Holter to a technician rather than an Einthoven. Early in the use of the technique we trusted too much in the reliability and especially the appropriateness of the automatic reading, but fortunately we no longer do so. Apart from the reading by the doctor himself, the technician should understand the anecdote, that is, the electrocardiographic event, correctly and should place it in its appropriate context; at least the beginning and the end, and even better, the whole tracing. It is only then that the phenomenon takes on its proper value and that its significance can really be understood. Herein are a few examples which, incidentally, are well addressed by the authors.

The authors insist that a ventricular premature beat should not be quantified and expressed in figures alone. How dearly we paid for these types of quantifications when we wanted rhythmology to be an exact science, until we realised that is not the number that reflects the gravity of the phenomenon but the morphology, the behaviour, and the context of the premature beats. We know now that the patient who is most at risk is not the one who has the most premature beats, and that the most appropriate medication for his or her treatment is not the one that suppresses the largest number. By "killing" premature beats (to use the English term "premature beat killer" applied for certain types of anti-arrhythmic drugs) we have killed too many patients in the not-too-distant past. Whatever the number that specifies a dangerous premature beat, it is not the exact number but its polymorphism, its absence of dependence on the sinus frequency, and even more its appearance in the context of exercise or ischemia.

Other examples? We have often proposed to palliate the difficulty in distinguishing the P waves on a Holter during tachycardia to help with special recordings, as, for instance, the oesophageal recordings. But these pseudoadvances did not come out of the laboratory because we know from clinical experience that the diagnosis is made on the first beats of the tachycardia and/or the last ones. As long as we know the beginning and the end of the story I do not recall any rhythmological diagnosis that would have been impossible on a Holter which would have been possible on a surface ECG consisting of the arrhythmia alone. The Holter report should not consist only of the 10 sec of the tracing necessary for the diagnosis of paroxysmal atrial fibrillation. It should also contain the end of the arrhythmia looking for the post-tachycardic pause, and as well for its beginning: not the last sinus beat but the last quarter of an hour or the last hour, which will only allow us to argue for an adrenergic or a vagal mechanism. This is not an electrophysiologist reflexion just curious of physiopathology, but the thought of a clinician who knows from experience that a beta-blocker will be successful in the first case and deleterious in the second.

To a picky reviewer who one day asked me, because I could not prove it, to remove a paragraph in an article in which I was formulating the concept that all cardiac rhythm troubles were related to the nervous autonomous system, I suggested reversing the burden of proof and for him to show me evidence of a single arrhythmia in which this system would not play a role. I had no trouble then in winning my case. However, to express such an opinion is no more difficult than to say that days alternate with nights. What is difficult is to explore the different modalities of a general situation giving convincing evidence. Holter recordings have favourably influenced the rhythmologists' thinking since the 1980s, at a time when they believed they had all the keys for their discipline through provocative methods. I am sure that the present manual will arouse a comprehensive understanding of the Holter technique, which at its beginning was too rooted by its accountant style of approach.

Chief Physician   Professor Philippe Coumel
Cardiology Department
Lariboisiere Hospital
Paris

Preface*

Long-term ECG recording has been known for some time but has recently been further developed owing to miniaturisation, digitalisation, and an increase in memory.

First of all, the newer techniques have improved the Holter method, which was first invented in the 1960s. Moreover, devices are currently being developed which can record ambulatory ECG for several days, and subcutaneous implanted loop recording devices can monitor the heart rhythm for more than a year. However, these event recorders only detect arrhythmic events that can be predefined in a very individualised manner.

Even with this progress in computerisation, indeed probably because of it, correct electrocardiographic interpretation remains the cornerstone for the accurate diagnoses that can be obtained through these very sophisticated methods.

We thought it useful to combine the quarter of a century of experience of one of us with the approach of a young cardiologist trained in the new time and era of modern cardiology, very focused on technology. Thereby we can offer the reader of this interpretation manual not only an explanation of the advantages of the method but also an understanding of its peculiarities and limits. As put explicitly in the title, we do not want to enter into the details of the indications and therapeutic proposals, but we do want to focus on the pure electrocardiographic diagnosis. There is already much literature on arrhythmias discovered via Holter recordings, but to use it properly one first has to be sure of the electrocardiographic diagnosis.

The long-term electrocardiographic recording, also known as ambulatory ECG recording was invented by Norman J. Holter at the beginning of the 1960s, and his name was given to this new diagnostic tool. Now under the name ECG Holter we imply a recording of all cardiac complexes for at least 24 hr. Its usefulness in the diagnosis of different arrhythmias and later in the diagnosis of myocardial ischemia, especially silent myocardial ischemia, has engendered a favourable technical evolution. It has led, on the one hand, to miniaturisation of the recording device itself and, on the other hand, to the provision of three leads, so that recording can take place without limitation during daily activities and night time sleep.

---

*See References 1–3, 6–8, 10, 13, 14, and 34.

At the same time, the reading devices started to become semiautomatic and sometimes even fully automatic to accelerate the reading and offer different calculations of the events.

In principle, there are two types of reading devices: The first requires a learning process during the first reading in order to distinguish between the wide ventricular complexes and the narrow supraventricular complexes for premature beats and tachycardia, as well as to eliminate artefacts. The device then remembers the criteria introduced during the first "learning" reading and does not stop on a complex which has already been analysed, so that the second reading is done in an automatically.

The second type takes an automatic reading based on ventricular complexes considered to be normal according to templates and registers all the others as abnormal. Nevertheless, the human reader may—or even better said *must*—verify the complexes judged by the machine to be normal in order to identify any that may actually be pathological and especially to eliminate artefacts. This second device seems to work faster at first, but once one takes the time to verify the complexes and the arrhythmias this is usually no longer the case.

The speed of the lecture depends firstly on the presence or absence of the different arrhythmias and even more on the quality of the tracing and its purity. An artefact is much more easily recognised by the experienced human eye than by an automatic reading device.

All reading devices ignore atrial activity and do not recognise the P wave. The presence and the relation of the P waves with the ventricular complexes remains the key for correct diagnosis of most arrhythmias, and this escapes the automatic reading device. The performance of the automatic reading depends on this. It is optimal for the premature ventricular beats, the ventricular tachycardia, and even supraventricular tachycardia, but cannot avoid the pitfall of an intraventricular aberration. All the other arrhythmias escape detection in an automatic reading.

A new generation of devices is now at our disposal. These are digitalised recorders with memory: there is no tape so no tape-related artefacts, such as an incorrect movement of the tape, are present. These recorders need very extensive memory storage because too much compression of the signal's graphic reproduction of the cardiac activity can alter the precision of the cardiac complex.

Contents

Chapter 1
Technical Aspects*

1.1 Recording

Optimal positioning of the electrodes is crucial if one is to wind up with a clean
recording of value, free of artefacts and parasites, for the entire run, especially
during periods of daily activity but also during sleep. One minute "lost" in placing
the electrodes is redeemed many times in time saved in the reading of the ECG
curves.

Figure 1.1 shows the recommended position of the seven electrodes for a three-
lead recording. The positioning can be modified if one wants to emphasise the signal
of the P waves or the ventricular complexes. In all cases, it is better to place the electrodes on the bones to avoid the electric potentials of the intercostal muscles. The
skin should be prepared methodically. Any chest hair must be shaved and the skin
must be degreased and even abraded if it is too thick. Even though the electrodes
are autoadhesive, additional fixation with hypoallergenic tape is mandatory to fix
the cable to the thorax and stabilise the system.

Movement of the cable owing to the patient's daily activities or during sleep is
often a source of artefacts, especially provoking movements of the baseline which
prevent correct interpretation of the ST segment.

There are various different electrodes at our disposal, but we have long preferred
the "Blue Sensor VL-00S-S, Medicotest, Denmark" electrode, which is made with a
special clip that prevents the transmission of the electrode's and thorax's movements
to the cable and vice-versa. The electrolyte placed in the electrode plays an important role in facilitating the contact between the electrode and the skin by diminishing
the impedance, so it is important to discard dry electrodes (or to add electrolyte gel).
After placing the electrodes on the skin, it is advisable to control the signal of each
derivation on an ECG strip.

---

*See References 6, 8, 10, 12, 13, 14, 16, 22, 33, and 34.

J. Adamec, R. Adamec, *ECG Holter*, DOI: 10.1007/978-0-387-78187-7_1,
© Springer Science+Business Media, LLC 2008

1

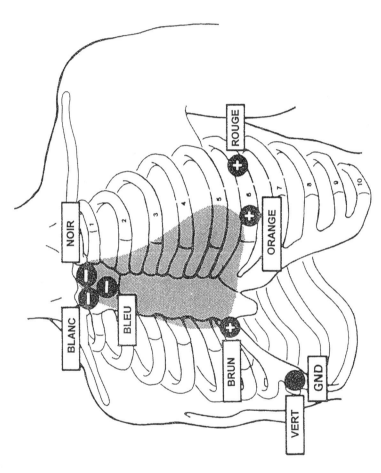

Fig. 1.1 Recommended position for the leads. These leads should be placed according to the international colour configuration. The green colour is the ground (GND)

1.2 Recorders

Recording devices have undergone rapid evolution and large magnetic bands have been replaced by tapes, decreasing the weight and volume. Digital recorders using memory chips have recently become even smaller and can be easily carried by the patient during daily activities.

1.3 Reading Systems

1.3.1 Manual Reading

Manual reading was developed by N. J. Holter. The ECG recorded continuously on a magnetic band was replayed on an oscilloscope screen superposing the ventricular complexes successively at accelerated speeds (120 to 240 times the normal speed). The normal sinus rhythm presented showed complexes aligned in a single picture with the premature beat appearing on one side and the pause on the other side of this alignment. Upon noting an anomaly, the operator stops the fast review and the ECG tracing appears on the screen enabling a diagnosis.

1.3.2 Semiautomatic Reading

Semiautomatic reading depends on the same principle of visualisation of the ventricular complexes aligned on the screen. During the first reading, the operator deals with the learning of the device. Selected criteria are programmed beforehand (prematurity, percentage, maximal frequency, pause duration, bradycardia, ST segment, artefacts, etc.), the device stops automatically with each abnormality, and the operator is asked to classify the anomaly. Once the anomaly is classified, it no longer stops the reading device but continues to be counted. The stops, quite frequent at the beginning of the run, become less and less frequent because the device stops only when a new anomaly appears. The visual control on the oscilloscope allows the operator to stop the reading at any point and to print the trace on ECG paper at the usual speed of 25 mm/s. Based on this learning, the device repeats the run, this time in a fully automatic mode which is based on the operator's classification and, at the same time, providing various numbers, calculations, statistics, diagrams, and figures. This semiautomatic reading technique will remain in use for a long period.

1.3.3 Automatic Reading

Automatic reading takes place without a learning phase, the device 'deciding' by itself which complex to consider as normal and which as pathological based on similarities with the templates.

At the end of this automatic reading, the device displays all the complexes considered to be normal and all the different types of those considered to be pathological, and the operator must then verify the selection.The device also provides a count of the events and statistics.

A fully automatic reading device with which there is no need for the operator to reinterpret the tracings looks promising at first glance because the automatic file contains many numbers, figures, and statistics, but all this accumulated data are not always correct and often do not reflect the truth. As the device is completely automatic, its interpretation value and efficiency diminish with the complexity of the recording. In our opinion, fully automatic recordings without a human superimposed access should be totally avoided.

1.3.4 Miniature Tracing

Some devices show a total impression of the miniaturised tracing (*full disclosure*) which actually represents the totality of the complexes but printed at an accelerated speed with a graphic compression. This allows us to look quickly for a specific symptomatic moment on the recording, but does not often give a precise diagnosis because of the compression and speed of the tracing.

1.3.5 Real-Time Interpretation

Reading in real time offers an analysis done at the moment of the recording with the help of microchips incorporated into the recording device which store the curves and, with the help of a dedicated program, classify and analyse the complexes as soon as they are detected and keep them in their memory according to this classification. However, as the device looks at the anomalies during the recording, misclassification cannot be corrected and there can only be validation.

1.4 Artefacts

Artefacts constitute Holter's Achilles' heel. They considerably complicate the reading, increase the length of the reading period, and sometimes confound the correct diagnosis. We must note and insist that most artefacts are better recognised by an experienced eye than by the computerised interpretation. In Holter cardiology the well-trained human specialist has not yet been replaced by a computer, and we are not yet in a chess game where "Deep Fritz" beats the world chess champion.

With each new artefact it is important to understand its origin and ideally be able to reproduce it. If the ECG tracing seems really unusual one should always consider that an artefact might explain the trace. If the artefact can be reproduced we avoid the trouble of looking for very rare unusual diagnoses. Enumerating all of the possible artefacts is virtually impossible because from time to time a new specimen appears to challenge the knowledge of the operator and the interpreter.

1.4.1 Artefacts Associated with the Recording

The ECG Holter recording should reflect the cardiac activity of normal daily life for each individual patient; sometimes we ask the patient to engage in even more activity on the day of the recording so that we can catch the anamnestic complaint on the tracing. Sweating as a result of physical activity is a major "enemy" of the electrodes. As noted earlier the best prevention is the care taken to place the electrodes with perfect skin preparation and careful fixing of the cable.

Artefacts that interfere completely with the reading of the curves are much less frequent today owing to the three leads; rarely will an artefact affect all three leads at once or affect them with the same intensity. Usually one of the leads can still provide the clue for a correct diagnosis (Fig. 1.2).

Thorax muscle contractions are often the source of artefacts, because they cause parasites that alter the baseline. As noted earlier, we fix the electrodes on the bony structures (ribs, sternum) to prevent artefacts from muscle activity. Static electricity owing to synthetic underwear can mimic pacemaker spikes.

1.4.2 Artefacts Associated with to the Recording Device

The tape recording can be influenced by artefacts owing to a rotation problem with the tape or by the tape itself. If the tape unwinds too slowly (very often because of battery problems—aged batteries or batteries exposed to the cold) a false "tachycardia" appears on the recording, whereas if the tape unwinds too fast a false "bradycardia" appears. However, if one looks carefully, the false tachycardia presents a "compression" of the complexes and of the PR or ST intervals. The false bradycardia presents widened complexes (Fig. 1.3).

Artefacts can also be due to an incompletely erased tape, reused after a previous recording. Even though the magnetic head should erase the previous tracing, it often does not do so completely because the position of the head is slightly different each time. To avoid this, it is important to fully erase the tape manually after each recording. Otherwise, we have a double recording, which can be mistaken for a tachycardia. Usually because one also finds the false complexes in the refractory period it does lead to the correct diagnosis. Fortunately, this is no longer a problem with digital recordings.

1.4.3 Artefacts Associated with Interpretation

Artefacts that are due to the reading devices are quite rare and depend on the specific device. These are the artefacts that cause the biggest problems with the automatic readings. A rare but intellectually interesting artefact is the reading of the tape backwards (Fig. 1.4).

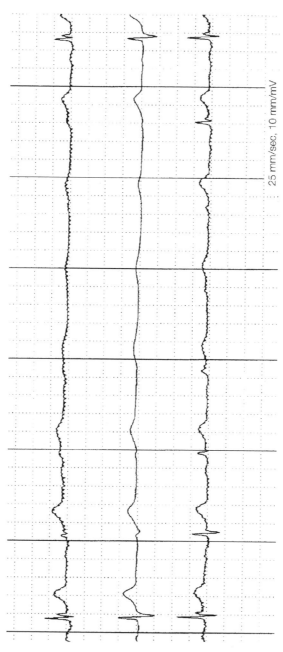

Fig. 1.2 The signal disappears completely on the first and second tracing. On the third tracing, the T waves persist and thus provide the clue for an artefact

25 mm/sec, 10 mm/mV

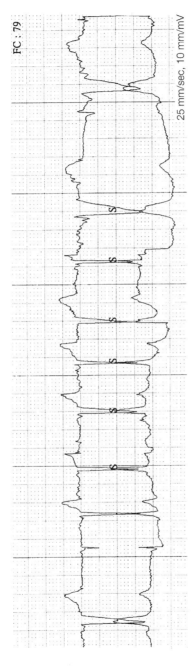

Fig. 1.3 The tape speed is incorrect. The first complex may be normal. Then we see a very narrow low-amplitude complex, and we think that the tape has stopped. The next complex is also compressed, as is the fourth complex. Three complexes that appear to be normal follow, and then once again a complex is compressed. The two last complexes are widened because the tape unwound faster than it should have

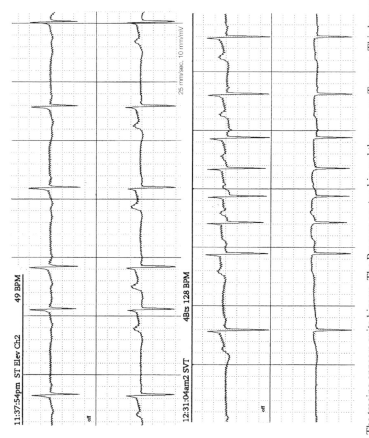

Fig. 1.4 (reproduced at 96 %). The tracing appears quite bizarre. The P waves are too big and there are no T waves. This happens when the tape is read in the reverse position "upside down." To get the correct reading, one has to turn the page upside down and then one sees a much more usual tracing with a sinus rhythm followed first by a premature supraventricular beat and then at the lower portion of the tracing an atrial tachycardia of 5 QRS

Chapter 2
Electrocardiographic Interpretation*

2.1 Peculiarities and Limits of ECG Holter Interpretations

The ECG Holter is recorded with one, two, or now with three *thoracic leads* that are *bipolar* and can thus record the electric potential difference between the positive and the negative electrodes. We are not referring here to thoracic leads (V) of the clinical 12-lead electrocardiogram because those are unipolar and record the difference between the potential of the thoracic electrode and Wilson's zero reference, despite many claims to the contrary by the producers of the different devices. Although some Holter leads may be similar to thoracic standard leads, especially to V5 or V1, they are not identical, and they do not allow us to determine the *axis in the frontal plane*. Consequently, none of the definitions based on the axis, as, for instance, the P sinus wave, are true in Holter recordings (see Sec. 4.2.1). This also explains why a *bundle branch* cannot be categorised and one may never know if one is in the presence of a right or left bundle branch block.

There are, however, *advantageous characteristics* that compensate for these limitations. It is essentially the *dynamic* of the recording, which is valuable for the diagnosis of sinoatrial and atrioventricular blocks, which enables us to visualise these and decide on the proper treatment. Moreover, the recording of the beginning and the end of the various paroxysmal tachycardias is a key factor for correct interpretation. The sinus function can often be deduced from the restarting of the sinus rhythm after the end of an atrial tachyarrhythmia (Fig. 2.1), and the revelation of silent myocardial ischemia also provides a prognostic factor. The dynamic of arrhythmias and especially the presence of intermittent atrial fibrillation or alternation between atrial fibrillation and atrial flutter often influence the therapeutics.

The following sections address these limitations and peculiarities in detail.

*See References 6, 9, 14, 16, 32, 33, and 34.

J. Adamec, R. Adamec, *ECG Holter*, DOI: 10.1007/978-0-387-78187-7_2,
© Springer Science+Business Media, LLC 2008

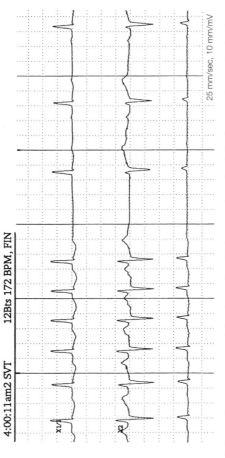

Fig. 2.1 At the beginning of the tracing we see an atrial tachycardia which stops abruptly. Only the second complex is of sinus origin, since it is preceded by a P wave of sinus morphology. The first complex following the tachycardia is of junctional origin

2.2 Basic Cardiac Rhythms

The diagnosis of the basic rhythm is essential. As the atrial activity is so important for its origin and as it cannot be recognised by the automatic evaluation of the reading device, it is up to the human to interpret it correctly. The basic rhythm may be the sinus rhythm during the whole recording, the sinus rhythm may alternate with one or different arrhythmias, or a specific arrhythmia may be the basic rhythm.

2.2.1 Sinus Rhythm

The impossibility of determining the axis of the P wave in the frontal plane precludes using the normal diagnostic criteria for the sinus rhythm as is done in the standard 12-lead electrocardiogram. Nevertheless, it is possible to deduce a sinus rhythm in the presence of repetitive positive P waves of identical morphology with a normal PR interval. A discrete variability in the frequency influenced by breathing and neurohumoral variations and progressive acceleration and deceleration indicate sinus rhythm. On the other hand, a "chronometric" regularity speaks more in favour of an ectopic origin. A sinus frequency below 40 bpm is indicative of a possible sinoatrial block. One must determine whether the slowing down of the rhythm was progressive (sinus bradycardia) or if the decrease in frequency was abrupt (sinoatrial block).

The acceleration of the sinus heart rate may reach the maximal heart rate determined by the patient's age (theoretical maximal heart rate). A heart rate frequency that is around or even exceeds the maximal theoretical heart rate strongly suggests a supraventricular tachycardia. With rapid heart rates, determining whether the onset was abrupt or not requires prolonged recordings. The automatic analysis of the arrhythmia by the device is very often confounded by these rapid heart rates because at these rates the premature onset of the supraventricular tachycardia represents only a minimal difference in the RR interval and thus cannot be recognised and correctly analysed by the automatic device.

2.2.2 Atrial Fibrillation

Atrial fibrillation is the second most usual basic rhythm. The fast atrial activity, irregular in its shape and chronology, is not always visible in a nonoptimal technical quality recording, in which case the diagnosis is essentially made on the irregular irregularity of the ventricular complexes. The presence of atrial fibrillation as the basic rhythm of the recording makes the electrocardiographic interpretation much more difficult because the appearance of the next ventricular complex cannot be foreseen.

Each regularity seen in the run of an atrial fibrillation has to be recorded and analysed. A regularity with a fast frequency and an identical ventricular morphology indicates junctional paroxysmal tachycardia, which may very well appear in the run of an atrial fibrillation. A regularity with a slow frequency indicates a junctional rhythm with a regular narrow QRS owing to an underlying complete atrioventricular block.

2.2.3 Atrial Flutter

The precise electrocardiographic diagnosis of *arterial flutter* is impossible because the morphology of the F waves should be judged from the DII, DIII, and aVF leads to find the characteristic morphology in addition to the negative preponderant appearanceand the left vectorial projection. Nevertheless, the regularity of the atrial activity at a frequency between 250 to 350 bpm with a typical aspect gives us the clue, especially if it is a type 1 flutter. The conduction to the ventricles is very often regular 2:1 or 3:1, but may vary. The ventricular activity then appears irregular but not irregularly irregular as in the atrial fibrillation. However, as in atrial fibrillation, it is impossible to predict exactly when the next ventricular complex, caused by the atrial activity, is due to appear.

During the same recording, atrial fibrillation and atrial flutter may be present intermittently. In this case, the correct diagnosis of atrial flutter is more difficult, especially if the flutter is of very short duration, because even during atrial fibrillation there may from time to time be an apparent intermittent coordination of the atrial activity. On the other hand, as soon as one notes irregular atrial activity followed by an irregular ventricular response, one must suspect a degeneration of atrial flutter into atrial fibrillation because the diagnosis of the latter is much more important for treatment and prognosis.

2.2.4 Atrial Tachycardia

Paroxysmal or permanent atrial tachycardia may as well represent the basic rhythm. Its diagnosis is not easy and should ideally be confirmed with a 12-lead clinical ECG; sometimes one must even add specific bipolar thoracic (Lewis) leads. On a Holter, it may be thought of as being in presence of ventricular activity that is either very regular without any of the variations suggesting a sinus rhythm or regularly irregular. In this last case, it usually presents itself with a ventricular activity coupled by two, with a constant ratio between the longest and the shortest distance between the ventricular couplets. This indicates an atrial heart rate more rapidly conducted to the ventricular level with a variable block, as, for instance, 2:1 or 3:1.

2.2.5 Ventricular Tachycardia

Ventricular tachycardia is much rarer as the basic rhythm, but if that is the case, it is a relatively slow tachycardia which lasts for the 24 hr of the recording without provoking hemodynamic alterations. It is also quite rare to have an *idioventricular-accelerated rhythm* as the basic rhythm. In both cases, one may find the atrial activity dissociated from the ventricular rhythm (it is much more visible during accelerated idioventricular rhythm because rarely does the ventricular heart rate exceed 100 bpm).

2.2.6 Atrial Silence

Occasionally an *atrial mutism*may be present. Ususally, in this case the ventricular rhythm is a junctional one. The differential diagnosis with an atrial fibrillation with very low atrial amplitude is difficult.

In the presence of a sinus rhythm complicated by an arrhythmia, it is better to interpret the ventricular complex during the sinus rhythm. If only arrhythmia is present during the recording, one must consider the origin of the arrhythmia itself in the interpretation of the ventricular complex.

2.3 Supraventricular Hyperexcitability

2.3.1 Supraventricular Premature Beats

Premature supraventricular beats appear on a Holter tracing as narrow QRS complexes, identical to the sinus complexes, but appearing earlier than when the next sinus complex is due. The automatic diagnosis of the premature supraventricular beat is based on the prematurity of the complex, which can be manually programmed, and on the supraventricular morphologic appearance of the complexes in that they are narrow. The device can count these premature supraventricular complexes, categorise them in hourly appearances, and present them graphically as well as in histograms. By definition a premature supraventricular beat that is not too premature, that is, less premature than the prematurity predefined by the device, can be ignored because the absence of the P wave or its slightly different aspect than the normal P wave is not recognised by the automatic interpretation system.

During visual human interpretation, the ectopic P wave is recognised and the origin of the premature beat can be determined as being of atrial origin. It is useful to compare the morphology of the repolarisation—meaning to look carefully at the ST segment and at the T wave, where the presence of an ectopic P wave in the same segment in the sinus rhythm where we are sure that no prematurity is present seems suspicious. The repetition of the suspicious segments increases the certitude of the presence of premature P waves.

The *atrial premature beats* may present the same charactreristics as on a clinical ECG. Nevertheless, the diagnosis of a multifocal atrial extrasystoly must to be made with caution because the polymorphism of the ectopic P waves may also be due to a change in the patient's position during recording (e.g., during sleep), provoked by the different projection of the atrial activity on the thoracic bipolar leads.

The *atrial extrasystolies* may be *blocked*, and in this case the differential diagnosis with sinus pauses may be difficult. To overcome the problem it is necessary to look carefully at the repolarisation phase of the previous complex. In principle, even if nothing indicates the hidden presence of an ectopic P wave in the ST-T segment, a blocked atrial premature beat cannot be altogether excluded because the low potential of the ectopic P wave may not modify the repolarisation of the QRS complex. Therefore, in some situations the possibility of blocked premature atrial beats must be considered in the explanation of a "sinus pause," even more so if the recording shows the simultaneous occurrence of premature atrial beats (Fig. 2.2).

Quantitative evaluation of the extrasystolies is of interest and may be useful in determining the cause of the extrasystoly. Nevertheless, it is important to remember that there is considerable variability from one recording to another.

Essentially, the *qualitative evaluation* represents the diagnosis of isolated extrasystolies, of bi- , tri- , and quadrigeminism of doublets or triplets. The last, by definition, represents supraventricular tachycardias. Extrasytoly repartition in the "nycthemer" leads us to suspect extrasystoly dependence on neurohumoral innervation. Prematurity during the active period of the day depends much more on the sympathic tone, whereas prematurity at the night depends on the vagal tone. It is also very useful to see if there is a correlation between the prematurity and the basic rhythm heart rate, in order to determine whether the prematurity appears during slow rhythm and disappears with acceleration of the rhythm, or if, on the contrary, the prematurity appears during a fast heart rate.

If we do not see any ectopic P wave before the narrow premature complex we are in the presence of a *junctional extrasystoly* and it is useful then to see whether or not there is retrograde conduction to the atrias, in which case we are observing atrial activity following the ventricular complex. This *retrograde atrial depolarisation* may alter the sinus activity and thus provoke an incomplete post-extrasystoly pause. Furthermore, this retrograde atrial activity, provoking an atrial contraction at the moment of the ventricular systoly, may (if the phenomenon persists long enough as, e.g., during bigeminism) become symptomatic, causing a clinical hypotension (the same phenomenon as in the pacemaker syndrome).

2.3.2 Supraventricular Tachycardia

By definition a supraventricular tachycardia consists of three consecutive premature beats, faster than 100 bpm, with a QRS complex identical to the sinus QRS. Using this definition, the device's automatic interpretation systemclearly recognises the supraventricular tachycardia. In regard to the premature beats, recognition of the tachycardia depends on the prematurity of the first complex and on the difference between the tachycardia's heart rate and the sinus heart rate. For this reason, a tachycardia appearing during a fast sinus rate may go undetected.

Using the figure of three premature complexes to determine a tachycardia is an arbitrary decision. The differential diagnosis of such a short supraventricular tachycardia is essentially an *interpolated supraventricular extrasystoly* followed by an isolated supraventricular extrasystoly. We are then in the presence of a sinus complex followed by three rapid complexes. This triad is usually detected by the automatic interpretation system and diagnosed as a supraventricular tachycardia. The electrocardiographic interpretation is not always easy because the atrioventricular conduction of the second sinus complex following the interpolated prematurity may be prolonged by the hidden conduction of the extrasystoly, and the sinus P wave

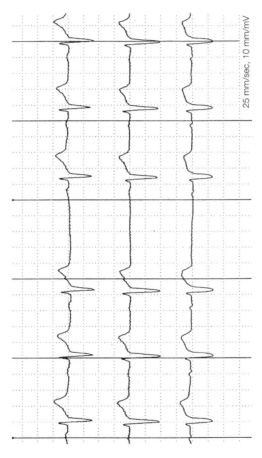

25 mm/sec, 10 mm/mV

Fig. 2.2 The pause on the tracing is in reality a post-premature beat pause owing to an atrial blocked premature beat. We see very clearly in the first and second tracing a notch in the ascending part of the T wave which hides a P wave

is not always seen clearly, as it is hidden in the T wave. An interpolated bigeminism may be mistaken for supraventricular tachycardias and it is then only the correct recognition of sinus P waves that can provide a clue and lead to the correct diagnosis (Fig. 2.3).

The discovery of ectopic P waves in a tachycardia run results in a much more precise diagonosis of its origin. The presence of more ectopic P waves than QRS complexes suggests a diagnosis of *more or less blocked atrial tachycardia* (Fig. 2.4). If the number of P waves is the same as the number of QRS complexes, one can make a differential diagnosis among an *atrial tachycardia with no block*, a *WPW*

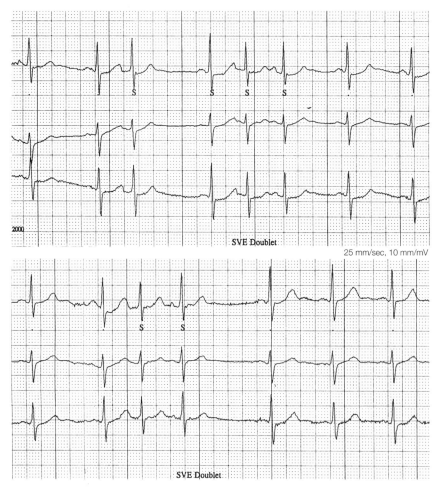

Fig. 2.3 In the upper part of the figure, the second complex is of sinus origin, followed first by a premature atrial beat and then by a pause. Between the fourth and sixth ventricular complex, we see an atrial premature interpolated beat. The last two complexes are of sinus origin. In the lower part of the figure, following the second complex, which is of sinus origin, we see a supraventricular doublet followed by a post-extrasystolic pause. The last three complexes are of sinus origin

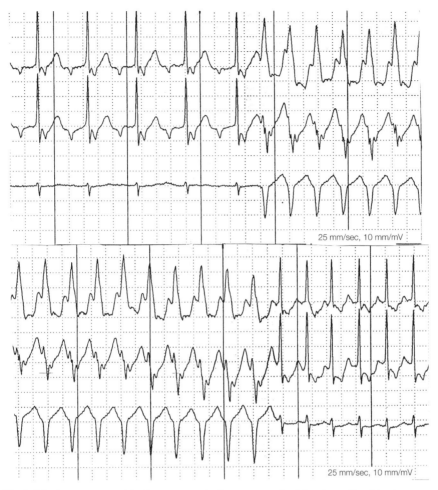

Fig. 2.4 In the upper part of the figure, we are in the presence of atrial tachycardia with a heart rate frequency of 175 bpm on the atrial level transmitted 2:1 to the ventricles. After the fifth ventricular complex, the conduction starts to be at 1:1, which provokes an intraventricular aberration. In the lower part of the figure, the 1:1 conduction is maintained with the persistence of the intraventricular aberration over ten complexes. Then, even though the conduction remains at 1:1, the aberration disappears and the ventricular complex becomes narrow

tachycardia, or an *AVNRT* (atrioventricular nodal-reentrant tachycardia). The position of the P wave close to the previous complex (the RP distance being shorter than the PR distance) indicates a diagnosis of an orthodromic WPW tachycardia in which the atrioventricular conduction follows the normal pathway using the AV node and the bundle. The retrograde conduction is the one that transits through the Kent bundle. An invisible P wave hidden in the previous QRS indicates an atrioventricular nodal-reentrant tachycardia. An atrial tachycardia without a block can have the P wave situated anywhere in the RR interval.

When describing a tachycardia it is important not to to forget to mention its frequency, the regularity of this frequency, its acceleration and deceleration, and the uniformity of the QRS complexes.

A narrow QRS tachycardia presents itself as a coupletseparated by short intervals, and a prolonged interval is usually provoked by more rapid atrial activity being transmitted irregularly to the ventricles with 3:2 or 4:3 conduction. It is then advisable to look very carefully at the intervals between the QRS complexes to see if there is rapid atrial activity, as, for instance, an atrial tachycardia with a block. It is essential to visualise the stops of the atrial tachycardia to assess the recovery of the sinus rhythm and quantify the time interval for its reappearance.

2.3.3 Atrial Fibrillation

The electrocardiographic diagnosis of *atrial fibrillation* is given by the presence of rapid atrial activity which is irregular (more than 400 bpm), with ventricular activity appearing with QRS complexes separated by RR intervals which are completely irregular.

Atrial fibrillation can be the basic rhythm or it may be present in episodes that are more or less prolonged which alternate with another basic rhythm, usually the sinus rhythm. In the first case the atrial fibrillation is present on the recording from the beginning to the end and in this form presents a difficulty for the automatic interpretation system to correctly identify the rhythm.

Sometimes, the atrial activity is not easily detected because its amplitude can be very small and thus hidden in the noise of the recording. On the other hand, this activity may have a very large amplitude, but evidence a regularity in its pattern, at least for a while, which may look like a flutter. In both cases the diagnosis is made on the basis of the irregular irregularity of the ventricular complexes.

Atrial fibrillation as the basic rhythm is complicated by the fact that we do not know in advance when the next QRS complex will appear. Therefore, in this case, the diagnosis of an aberration in the intraventricular conduction and fusion is difficult.

It is useful to establish the atrial fibrillation's heart rate in order to recognise the highest and lowest heart rates during rest (sleep) and during various activities of daily life (Fig. 2.5). An atrial fibrillation which remains rapid during the night and does not present nycthemeral slowing suggests in the first instance hyperthyroidism. We must think also of conditions that provoke a high catecholamine level as, for example, an anaemia or a cardiac insufficiency. On the other hand, a slowing in the atrial fibrillation may hide an intermittent complete atrioventricular block and the only way to make the correct diagnosis is to look for ventricular regularity that is present for a more-or-less extended period. Based on the irregularity (the definition of atrial fibrillation), the discovery of two identical RR intervals with slow heart rates leads us to diagnose an intermittent atrioventricular block with the appearance of an escape rhythm.

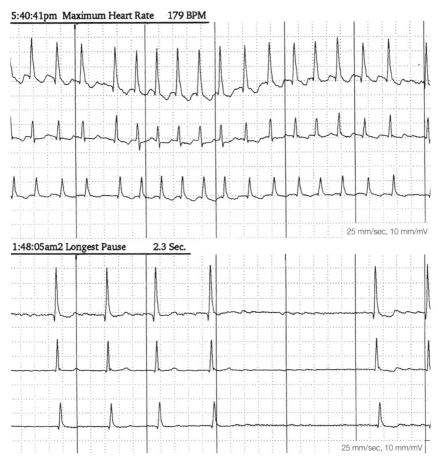

Fig. 2.5 (reproduced at 96%). The upper part of the figure shows a maximal cardiac heart rate of atrial fibrillation around 200 bpm. In the lower part of the figure (same patient, but during night), the heart rate falls and so pauses may appear. There is a pause of 2.3 sec, which reflects the atrioventricular conduction

In principle, pauses in atrial fibrillation reflect the state of the conduction at the atrioventricular level, especially at the site of the node. Paradoxically, some pauses may be induced by a very rapid heart rate of the atrial fibrillation, which provokes a "sideration" of the atrioventricular node.

The atrial fibrillation may be a *paroxysmal* fibrillation, appearing once or a few times during the 24-hr electrocardiographic recording. These paroxysmal episodes may occur at any moment of the recording. It is very useful to note the exact time of their occurrence because some paroxysmal atrial fibrillations appear during the "vagal" periods and others during the "sympathic" periods.

Atrial fibrillation of vagal origin appears during the periods influenced by the vagal tone, especially at night, during the early hours of the dawn, and after eating. The onset of paroxysmal episodes is usually during the slowing of the basic sinus rhythm or after an episode of atrial premature beats, often in bigeminism (Fig. 2.6). Once the atrial fibrillation, even from vagal onset, is established it may become rapid, may last for a long period of time, and may actually continue during the sympathic tone period.

Atrial fibrillation of sympathic origin usually appears during the acceleration of the basic sinus rhythm, often during physical exercice or in the presence of psychological stress.

It is very important to visualise the cessation of the atrial fibrillation in order to evaluate the time necessary for the sinus rhythm to reappear. This period may be assimilated in the *sinus recovery time*, which is determined in endocavitory electrophysiological procedures (EEP) to evaluate the sinus function. It is less easy to correct it according to the previous frequency of the arrhythmia because the recovery time also depends on the length of the arrhythmia itself and not only on its heart rate. Thus even if it may not be considered as a strict equivalent of the sinus recovery time, a delayed recovery of the sinus function (more than 3 sec) is nevertheless a very useful argument in favour of a *sick sinus syndrome* (Fig. 2.7).

It is very difficult to diagnose correctly very short onsets of atrial fibrillation (fewer than nine complexes) because even onsets of supraventricular tachycardias present a certain irregularity, the onset often being rapid and the basal line not taking account of the distinction. Therefore we must remain cautious regarding these very short episodes before calling them atrial fibrillation, especially because of the therapeutic consequences, as, for instance, a decision to treat for anticoagulation. On the other hand, to recognise very short episodes of sinus rhythm in atrial fibrillation is very important because it changes the therapeutic attitude drastically: the issue is not to cardiovert but to maintain the sinus rhythm (Fig. 2.8).

An *intraventricular conduction aberration* (Ashman phenomenon) is a quite frequent phenomenon and expresses itself with the appearance of a right delay morphology. The right bundle branch block may be more or less complete. A left delay (left bundle branch block morphology) is also possible but less usual. It is not always easy to make the correct differential diagnosis between this phenomenon and premature ventricular beats or short onsets of ventricular tachycardias. To render the correct diagnosis, it is important to look not only at the prematurity of the complex (which means the distance from the previous narrow complex) but to measure the duration of the previous diastoly. The correct diagnosis is important because one must distinguish between an intraventricular conduction aberration and nonsustained ventricular tachycardias (Fig. 2.9). It is often necessary to have long recordings at one's disposal in order to be able to correctly assess the wide QRS complex dependence on the heart rate frequency.

Sometimes the impossibility of distinguishing between the two on the Holter recording forces us to perform a stress test, where it is easier to fix a specific ventricular heart rate and the dependence of the wide QRS on the cardiac frequency may become more obvious. The appearance of this *phase 3 bundle branch block*

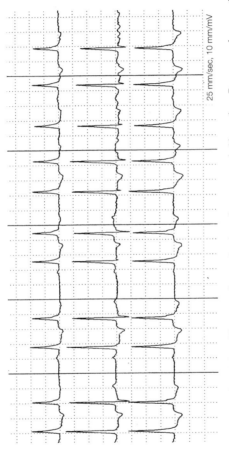

25 mm/sec, 10 mm/mV

Fig. 2.6 Normal sinus rhythm with atrial bigeminism. The seventh complex is no longer preceded by a sinus P wave, and we see the onset of paroxysmal atrial fibrillation

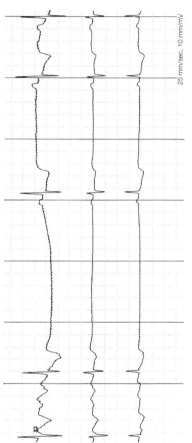

25 mm/sec; 10 mm/mV

Fig. 2.7 On the left of the tracing we see an atrial fibrillation which suddenly stops, followed by a pause of nearly 3 sec, followed by the appearance of a sinoatrial 2:1 block; only then, on the right side of the tracing (last ventricular complex of the tracing) does the normal sinus rhythm appear. The presence concomitantly of fast arrhythmia (atrial fibrillation) with sinus dysfunction (pause of nearly 3 sec) and a sinoatrial block indicates a sick sinus syndrome

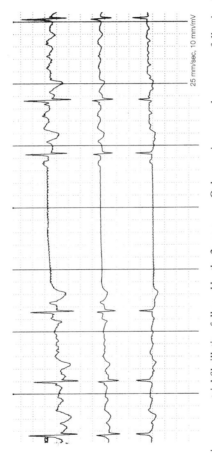

25 mm/sec, 10 mm/mV

Fig. 2.8 On the left of the tracing we see atrial fibrillation followed by the 2 sec pause. Only one sinus complex appears, following the pause, but the fibrillatory activity reappears in its repolarisation phase

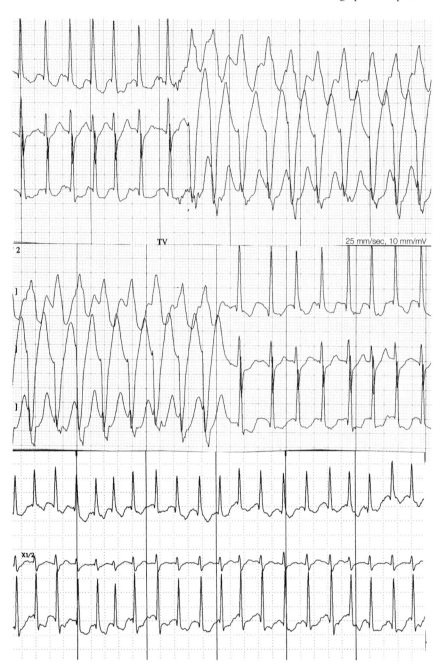

Fig. 2.9 (reproduced at 96.5%). We see a fast atrial fibrillation with some regular sequences appearing with a wide QRS. The whole page belongs to the same patient. The differential diagnosis is between a phase 3 aberration and and nonsustained ventricular tachycardia. In the upper part of the figure, the ventricular complexes appear faster; in the middle, there are some narrower ventricular complexes (indicating a fusion phenomenon), which is an argument for a ventricular origin; in the lower part we see that even for a faster heart rate frequency, the complex remains narrow. We can thus conclude that the atrial fibrillation is complicated by a ventricular tachycardia

even though it is frequency dependent is not strictly fixed, and the frequencies with which the block appears and disappears are not exactly the same. We are not in the presence of a cut-off point but rather in a grey area where this aberration may appear and disappear. In addition to the Ashman phenomenon to correctly diagnose a ventricular tachycardia in the presence of atrial fibrillation, one lacks the notion of atrioventricular dissociation. The fusion phenomenon is not easy to determine either because of the uncertainty of the appearance of the next ventricular complex.

Every noted regularity in atrial fibrillation indicates the presence of another arrhythmia. This regularity may be rapid, involving the coupling time of a supraventricular or ventricular premature complex, and may present as a bi-, tri- , or quadrigeminism or as doublets. Even a supraventricular tachycardia may be present in the middle of an atrial fibrillation because the junction does not belong to the atrial fibrillation arrhythmic substrate. The junction may cause a tachycardia, and if it is faster than the atrial fibrillation it may dominate the ventricle activation (the atrias cannot be activated in atrial fibrillation). Ventricular tachycardia may, of course, appear during atrial fibrillation. Sometimes, as discussed earlier, the correct diagnosis may be difficult as it is not easily distinguished from an intraventricular aberration conduction phenomenon (Fig. 2.10).

The regularity may be slowand then one has to think in terms of a complete atrioventricular block causing the appearance of a substitute rhythm, either junctional or ventricular. The atrial fibrillation continues to dominate the atrias but the ventricles are activated by an escape rhythm. It may be an escape single complex or a rhythm more or less extended, depending on the duration of the atrioventricular block.

2.3.4 Atrial Flutter

The diagnosis of atrial flutter on a 12-lead Holter recording is in principle impossible because one needs the "true" 12-lead electrocardiogram and especially the DII , DIII, aVF leads . Nevertheless one may consider such a diagnosis in the presence of fast atrial activity that is regular with a "dents de scie" character and is conducted to the ventricular level in a regular ratio—usually 2:1 but possibly 3:1, 4:1, or more. It may also have an irregular character when different ratios alternate in sequence, but one always finds a regular pattern in the apparent irregularity. Rarely it may be a 1:1 ratio and then we speak of an *unblocked atrial flutter*, which then provokes a very rapid ventricular conduction. The atrial activity heart rate is usually around 250 to 350 bpm; the slower heart rate is usually found in long-duration flutters and in flutters influenced by therapeutic measures, as, for instance, in treatment with amiodarone (Fig. 2.11).

The *first differential diagnosis* to consider is the atrial fibrillation. Often in atrial fibrillation, one recognises an atrial activity which becomes more or less regular and presents a larger amplitude. But the regularity has to persist for a long time before one can diagnose an atrial flutter. We must note that these two arrhythmias are very often associated on a 24-hr tracing. Therefore we may find a basic rhythm in atrial fibrillation with bouts of atrial flutter and, on the other hand, find runs of atrial

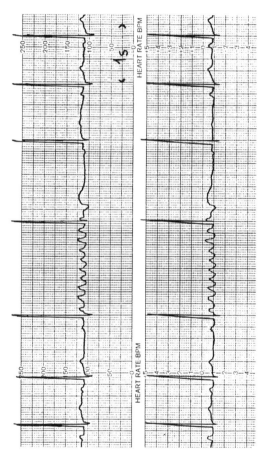

Fig. 2.10 In the middle of the tracing we see a bizarre image with a fast atrial activity heart rate of about 350 bpm, which indicates an atrial flutter. This activity is present only during one cardiac revolution, extending the RR interval. We then see a QRS complex preceded by an ectopic P wave. The last two complexes are once more of sinus origin

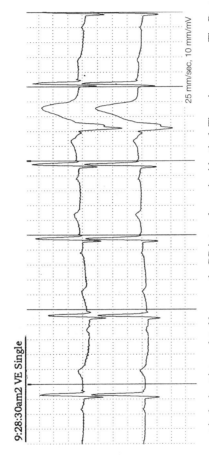

Fig. 2.11 We see a premature ventricular beat interpolated because the RR interval remains identical. There is no pause. The P wave of the complex following the premature beat is hidden in the T wave of the extrasystoly (concealed conduction)

fibrillation in the presence of chronic atrial flutter. Recognising and differentiating the two rhythms is important because of the therapeutic implications; the success rate for recognition of an overdrive (fast atrial stimulation) or ablation is lower if the flutter alternates with atrial fibrillation. The decision to anticoagulate is also influenced by an accurate interpretation of the arrhythmias involved.

The second arrhythmia to consider in the differential diagnosis is the *atrial tachycardia with block* (tachysystoly with block). The absence or presence of the isoelectric line is relatively unimportant as its morphology does not help much on the Holter recording. It is the atrial frequency that provides the clue. The atrial tachycardia with block (tachysystoly) usually has an atrial heart rate that does not exceed 270–280 bpm. It is true that an atrial flutter may have such slow atrial activity but the atrial F waves are usually quite visible.

The *intraventricular aberration* that appears as a phase 3 block may also be seen in the presence of atrial flutter and in that case the diagnosis may be tricky. Nevertheless, even though in the presence of atrial flutter the arrival of the next ventricular complex is uncertain; it may occur only in a well determined interval in accordance with the 1:1, 2:1, 3:1, etc, ratio . This facilitates the correct diagnosis. The Wenkebach phenomenon modifying the atrioventricular conduction is present only rarely. It is seen more frequently in the conduction of the atrial tachycardia with block (tachysystoly), which is responsible for a ventricular irregular response.

2.4 Ventricular Hyperexcitability

2.4.1 Ventricular Premature Beats

The *premature ventricular beats* are the most easily detected on a Holter recording by the automatic interpretation system because the initial diagnosis is based on the prematurity of the complex, as well as on its appearance, which differs from the sinus QRS especially in its width. For this reason, the diagnosis of ventricular premature beats is very precise and may be altered only by presence of parasites or artefacts. But we must bear in mind that no automatic interpretation can differentiate between a true premature ventricular beat and a supraventricular premature beat with an aberration.

The detection of ventricular premature beats easily discloses many of their aspects as the point-by-point detection analyses the whole ventricular complex and its full morphology. Obviously, however, as the sinus ventricular complex changes its appearance during the recording owing to the fact that the patient engages in different activities and episodes of sleep, the premature ventricular beats may also present differently.

Ventricular premature detection discloses different aspects of these premature beats because the system looks at all the anomalies and ventricular complex morphologies point by point. Since the ventricular complex in sinus rhythm already presents variations, either in form or in appearance during the recording owing to the fact that it is done while the patient is engaging in daily activities and spending hours in sleep, the premature ventricular beats may also present differences during the recording, and the automatic interpretation system produces numerous forms. Therefore we are clearly seeing a polymorphism of the ventricular prematurity and it is important to reassess all of the types observed to ensure that they are real rather than a result of the full automatic interpretation. Prematurity is one of the essential elements for the correct diagnosis, the belated ventricular premature beats (R/P) may escape the automatic diagnosis, particularly if they are really delayed and there is a fusion phenomenon between the premature ventricular beat and the following sinus complex. These factors result in a narrowing of the ventricular complex, which makes its recognition by the automatic interpretation system even more problematic.

The *quantitative diagnosis* is usually strongly supported by automatic interpretation as well as by numerisation of the bi- and trigeminism. The hourly expression and the graphic representation are useful for determining the dependence of the ventricular prematurity on the neurovegetative system. The prematurity that manifests itself essentially during the daytime hours is considered to be of catecholaminic origin, whereas the prematurity that appears at night when the heart rhythm is slower is thought to be of vagal origin.

A prematurity which maintains itself during the 24-hr recording is a ventricular hyperexcitability that does not depend on the neurovegetative system, and its origin must be reassessed.

The *qualitative diagnosis* depends in the first instance on the prematurity uniformity or its polymorphism. The polymorphism must always be considered with caution as must the automatic evaluation, as we discussed earlier. It is also important that the operator confirm that it is a true polymorphism suggestive of a polytropism of the extrasystoly. The variant appearance of the extrasystoly must be analysed bearing in mind the different aspects of the basic rhythm, for instance, the sinus rhythm. If an extrasystoly seems different, but the basic rhythm also presents modifications of its morphology, the difference with the extrasystoly is quite virtual. We must not forget that the recording is done when the patient is in different positions and that the morphology appears differently in standing, sitting, or lying down positions. The measure of the coupling time may help because an identical coupling time tells against a different origin of the complex. Nevertheless, we must note that the vagal frequency may modify coupling time. Bi-, tri, and quadrigeminism are easily diagnosed on the recording. This phenomenon is very often dependent on the frequency of the basic rhythm .

The *interpolated ventricular extrasystolies* present a diagnostic problem (Fig. 2.11), in particular if the ventricular complex of the basic rhythm following the extrasystoly presents an intraventricular conduction aberration, which is a quite frequent occurrence. In this case, the automatic interpretation may lead to a false diagnosis of ventricular tachycardia of three complexes or, rarely, misinterpret an interpolated extrasystoly with a bigeminism for a nonsustained ventricular tachycardia. We must always look very carefully for P waves and once there is evidence of concealed conduction we can make the correct diagnosis. These runs often have a polymorphic or bimorphic morphology, and this is in contradistinction to the runs of ventricular tachycardia, which are usually monomorphic.

2.4.2 Ventricular Tachycardia

The ventricular tachycardia is by definition a sequence of three wide ventricular complexes with heart rate frequencies of more than 100 bpm, and the first complex must be premature . The distinction between a sustained and a nonsustained tachycardia is arbitrary and was determined to be 30 sec. The ventricular tachycardia in its sustained appearance is usually not very difficult to diagnose by the automatic interpretation system. The *differential diagnosis* is a supraventricular tachycardia with an intraventricular conduction aberration with either a right or a left delay. The second differential diagnosis is a WPW syndrome tachycardia with an antidromic access (the conduction to the ventricles is over the accessory pathway).

The *quantitative diagnosis* of ventricular tachycardia is also very well interpreted by the automatic device, which gives both the repartition of the tachycardia in the nycthemeral cycle and hourly histograms. In the same way as for the premature ventricular beats, the presentation of the ventricular tachycardia may have particularities that escape the automatic interpretation and may be interpreted as polymorphisms. Therefore, it is always useful to compare the tachycardia to the normal basic rhythm and especially to look at the purest morphology of the tachycardia in comparison with the one of the basic rhythm. The tachycardia frequency is a useful element not only for expressing the maximal heart rate of the tachycardia but, equally important, for determining if the tachycardia accelerates during its run or if, on the contrary, it decelerates.

The *repartition* of the ventricular tachycardia during the day may be indicative of the presence or absence of the influence of the neurovegetative system. The ventricular tachycardias which manifest themselves essentially during the daytime, especially in the early hours of the morning, are thought to be influenced by the catecholamines; on the other hand, the tachycardias which occur at night may be influenced by the vagus, either directly or by slowing down the heart rate frequency. The correct analyses of the ST segment preceding the tachycardia may reveal a possibly silent ischemia, which may be its cause. However, as we will see in Sec. 4.7.2 the correct diagnosis of a silent ischemia is quite difficult on a 24-hr Holter recording.

2.4.3 Differential Diagnosis of a Wide QRS Tachycardia

A supraventricular tachycardia can have a wide QRS ventricular complex provoking a false aspect of *bundle branch block*. On a 24-hr Holter recording it is not easy to distinguish this supraventricular tachycardia with intraventricular conduction aberration from a true ventricular tachycardia (Figs. 2.12 and 2.13).

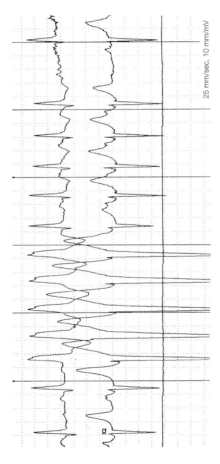

25 mm/sec, 10 mm/mV

Fig. 2.12 After the second sinus complex, we see the onset of a wide QRS tachycardia with a heart rate frequency of about 170 bpm. The tachycardia progressively slows down and after five complexes, the heart rate is only around 150 bpm and the QRS complex becomes narrow. At the end, the heart rate of the tachycardia is even slower, being at 130 bpm. We are observing an atrial tachycardia, which at the beginning presented a conduction aberration. If the tachycardia had stopped during the wide QRS complexes (meaning before the sixth complex), based on this tracing we could have falsely considered this tachycardia as being of ventricular origin

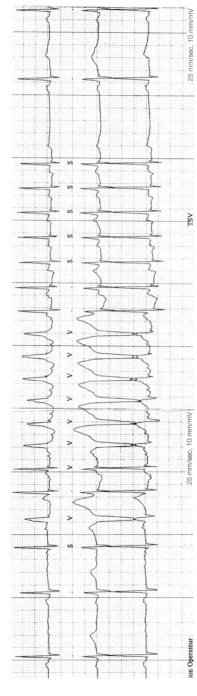

Fig. 2.13 An example of a tachycardia which is a differential diagnosis between a ventricular tachycardia and a supraventricular tachycardia with aberration. On the left of the tracing, we see two sinus complexes followed first by a premature atrial beat and then by a wide QRS complex preceded by an ectopic P wave. Owing to the ectopic P wave, we know we are in the presence of intraventricular conduction aberration. The next two QRS are narrow. Then follow six complexes of a wide QRS which have the same morphology as the second complex. We find a P wave equidistant between each two QRS. The access finishes with seven complexes with narrow QRS, indicating that we are in the presence of atrial tachycardia with intermittent aberration. A second way to explain this tracing would be to consider a double tachycardia from atrial and ventricular origin at the same time, but this seems to be less likely

The following points can help in making a differential diagnosis:

(a) *QRS duration*: the wider the QRS, the more certain its ventricular origin. A QRS duration of more than 140 msec speaks strongly in favour of ventricular origin.

(b) *QRS morphology*: a monomorphous morphology, in particular a wide QS, speaks strongly in favour of a ventricular origin as does a very notched QRS not having the first big deflexion very early, which means sooner than 100 msec.

(c) *Tachycardia speed*: a wide QRS tachycardia presenting quite a slow frequency (between 100 and 140 bpm) is usually of ventricular origin because it would be very unusual at this quite slow heart rate for a supraventricular tachycardia to present an aberration (Fig. 2.14).

(d) *Tachycardia onset*: a tachycardia which starts in the way that its first complex is only very slightly premature indicates a ventricular origin because it is difficult to imagine that an aberration has already taken place.

(e) The presence of *atrioventricular dissociation* indicates a ventricular origin of the tachycardia. Nevertheless, it is not easy to find a dissociation on a Holter recording because we have only two or three leads at our disposal and not the 12 leads of a normal surface electrocardiogram. Moreover, the ECG Holter is quite frequently altered by parasites and artefacts. Thus, the atrioventricular dissociation is less useful for the correct diagnosis of ventricular tachycardia on a Holter recording than on a standard 12-lead electrocardiogram.

(f) The presence of *a narrow QRS tachycardia* (of supraventricular origin) on another moment of the recording speaks in favour of supraventricular origin of the wide QRS tachycardia if the wide QRS tachycardia is shorter than the narrow supraventricular QRS tachycardia and if at its onset the latter presents a transitory intraventricular aberration.

We must always be very cautious before diagnosing a ventricular tachycardia because this diagnosis has implications for important prognostic consequences and therapeutic measures. If the electrocardiographic recording is not good enough to be sure of the diagnosis it is preferable to use the term *wide QRS tachycardia* and leave it to the clinician who knows the patient to put this diagnosis into the correct clinical context. Unfortunately, very often, the reader of the Holter recording is not well informed as to the clinical situation and this is the moment to emphasise that the best Holter interpretations are made by the cardiologists who have seen the patient clinically, examined him or her, and are also able to read the ECG Holter and interpret the tracings correctly. Ventricular origin is very seriously considered in a coronary patient who has ever had a myocardial infarction.

2.4.4 Accelerated Idioventricular Rhythm (AIVR)

The decision to take the heart rate frequency of 100 bpm to distinguish between a ventricular tachycardia (>100 bpm) and AIVR (<100 bpm) is too arbitrary. This simplistic definition does not take elementary elements into account and does not

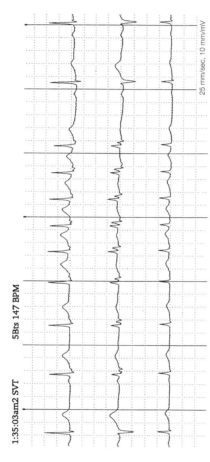

Fig. 2.14 The first complex is a sinus complex. Following the second sinus P wave, we see the appearance of a wide complex, clearly visible in the second lead but seeming falsely to be narrow in the first and third leads. Then we have seven identical complexes, and an accelerating heart rate frequency: 80 bpm at the beginning and 140 bpm at the end. The wide morphology appears slowly in the second lead. In the first lead, we see quite a wide notched S wave (giving a false aspect of a retrograde P wave), but in this lead, the width is not obvious. In the upper left corner of the figure, we can see that the automatic reading was confounded in that it considered the tachycardia to be a supraventricular tachycardia of five QRS. The correct interpretation is a ventricular tachycardia of eight QRS. Thus the machine was fooled not only about the origin of the tachycardia but about its duration as well

recognise an ectopic tachycardia. The latter starts with a prematurity such as an extrasystoly and finishes with a pause similar to the post-extrasystoly pause and an accelerated idioventricular rhythm, which, because it is faster than the sinus rhythm, dominates the latter. Therefore it is logical to consider as ventricular tachy-cardias even tachycardias that are slower than 100 bpm but which keep the basal characteristics of an ectopic tachycardia. In addition, a ventricular tachycardia can be slowed down below 100 bpm in the presence of different medications, as, for example, amiodarone. Figure 2.14 documents the simplistic approach based only on the heart rate frequency. The ventricular tachycardia starts with a frequency of 80 bpm (AIVR?) and terminates with a heart rate frequency of 140 bpm.

It is always advisable to quantify the speed of the tachycardia exactly and this is one way of showing that we are considering elements other than the heart rate for its definition. As can be seen in the example in the Fig. 2.14, there are tachycardias that are below 100 bpm.

2.5 Pauses and Bradycardia

2.5.1 Generalities

All reading devices ignore the P wave. For this reason, the bradycardia is revealed to the automatic reading device as a bradycardia of the ventricular complexes and the duration of the pause is measured between two successive ventricular complexes. We consider every ventricular heart rate equal to or less than 50 bpm as *bradycardia*, but this can be modified by the programming of the device. The automatic reader considers a *pause* to be equal to or longer than 2 sec or twice the distance of the previous RR interval.

2.5.2 Sinus Bradycardia

Sinus bradycardia is a bradycardia where each ventricular complex is preceded by a P wave of sinus morphology (see Sec. 4.2.1) with a heart rate frequency of 50 bpm or less.

The Holter recording allows us to visualise the slowing of the heart rate frequency that leads to the bradycardia and thus enables us to distinguish between a true sinus bradycardia, where the slowing down is progressive, and different forms of sinoatrial block, where the slowing is much more abrupt depending on the degree and the specificity of the block. The sinus bradycardia may be the result of vagal hyperstimulation and at this stage it usually presents with a PR interval at the upper limit of normal or even with a first-degree atrioventricular block. The isolated sinus bradycardia is more an expression of the dysfunction of the sinus node and the PR remains relatively short for the heart rate frequency.

Some medications may lead to sinus bradycardia as, for instance, digoxine, certain antiarrhythmics, especially beta-blockers or amiodarone. One must always be cautious when the patient uses eye drops.

2.5.3 False Sinus Bradycardia

False sinus bradycardia is relatively common and is frequently not interpreted correctly by the automatic reader. It is a bradycardia which may be caused by atrial bigeminism, where very often the atrial premature beats remain blocked (Fig. 2.15). As the ectopic P waves are very often not very well seen or not seen at all, the diagnosis is not an easy one.

In case of doubt, it is important to compare carefully the repolarisation segment (ST-T) of a ventricular complex suspected of hiding a blocked atrial premature beat with a complex where a premature beat cannot be (this means a complex out of the bradycardic pattern). An irregularity in the morphology or a notch, especially if repeated in the bradycardia, is an argument for the hidden prematurity. The presence of atrial premature beats conducting to the ventricle speaks in favour of this diagnosis as does the bradycardia's rapid and sudden appearance and disappearance.

2.5.4 Atrioventricular Bradycardia

The *atrioventricular (AV) bradycardia* depends on the degree and the frequency of the escape rhythms. The *second-degree atrioventricular block of type 1 and type 2* are very rarely responsible of an important bradycardia. The *2:1 atrioventricular block or the atrioventricular block of advanced degree* may lead to a bradycardia which is modified by the escape rhythm. In the same way, in presence of a *complete atrioventricular block*, the heart rate frequency depends of the escape rhythm.

2.5.5 Sinus Dysfunction

Pauses as an expression of sinus dysfunction usually appear at the end of atrial tachycardias, especially at the end of atrial fibrillation. The automatic reading devices, ignoring the atrial activity, do recognise the ventricular pause and they actually measure the distance between the last ventricular complex of the tachycardia and the first ventricular complex of the rhythm that appears after the end of the tachyarrhythmia. This does not always correspond to a sinus pause because the arrhythmia at the atrial level may persist after the last ventricular complex and it is not always a sinus rhythm that appears after the arrhythmia has stopped; the sinus pause expands until the appearance of the first P wave of sinus origin. Sometimes one cannot determine the moment of the recovery of the sinus rhythm because either a junctional or an atrial rhythm appearing beforehand prevented the appearance of the sinus rhythm (Figs. 2.16 and 2.17).

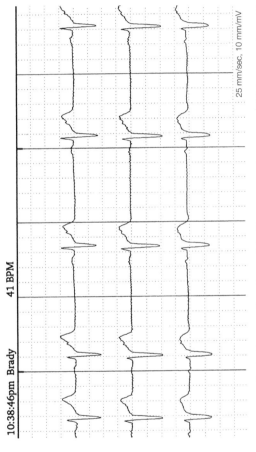

Fig. 2.15 Following the second sinus complex in the ascending phase of the T wave, a notch appears which is a premature atrial beat and it remains blocked. The same event is noted on the following three complexes. These four premature atrial blocked beats provoke a false bradycardia with a heart rate around 40 bpm. On the first complex we do not see notching on the T wave, which confirms the presence of the notch, due to the blocked atrial premature beats on the following complexes

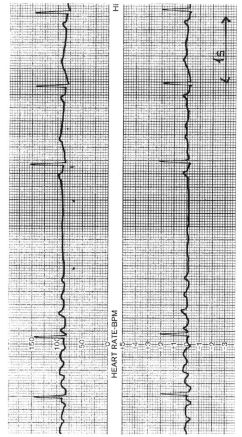

Fig. 2.16 We see the disappearance of an atrial fibrillation and the appearance of a sinus rhythm. The first two complexes are due to the atrial fibrillation, which continues on the atrial level following the second ventricular complex. The three last complexes that follow the pause are of sinus origin. If we measure the ventricular pause as the automatic recording and interpretation systems do, it lasts up to 2.6 sec. However, its duration is overestimated by the automatic device, because the correct way to measure it is between the last atrial activity signal and the P wave. Therefore, the correct measure is only 1.8 sec, which does not suggest sinus dysfunction. If we had considered only the automatic device interpretation, we might have considered a sick sinus syndrome, but there are no clear-cut arguments for it on this tracing

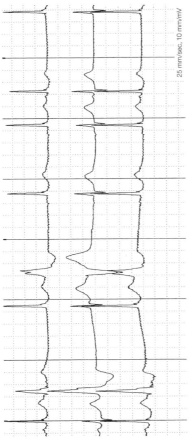

25 mm/sec, 10 mm/mV

Fig. 2.17 The first sinus complex is followed by a premature beat with a wide QRS and a retrograde conduction. We then see a pause that ends with a narrow QRS which is not preceded by a P wave, followed by the same premature beat with a wide QRS. Following the pause, we see two narrow complexes that are not of sinus origin, the second one being followed by an atrial premature beat. We can imagine that the first premature beat (the second QRS on the tracing) with its retrograde P wave paralyses the sinus function, which remains invisible for the rest of the tracing, so we can consider a sinus dysfunction

2.5.6 Post-Premature Atrial Blocked Beat

The *pause provoked by blocked atrial premature beat* is a post-extrasystolic pause but the atrial extrasystoly is not always visible. Sometimes, there may be more than one extrasystoly—as, for example, a blocked doublet or even a short shred of atrial tachycardia or blocked atrial tachycardia which extends the ventricular pause.

2.5.7 Bradycardia during Atrial Fibrillation

A *bradycardia during atrial fibrillation* indicates a conduction problem at the level of the atrioventricular node. The appearance of a regular bradycardia implies the appearance of a transitory complete atrioventricular block and the bradycardia is then an escape rhythm (junctional if the QRS is narrow, or identical to the fibrillation). When it is permanent the complete atrioventricular block manifests with a fast irregular atrial activity and a regular ventricular escape rhythm that is often slow. Pauses in the middle of atrial fibrillation express atrioventricular (AV) conduction. Bradycardia during atrial flutter is also an expression of the atrioventricular conduction. The appearance of a complete atrioventricular block during atrial flutter is difficult, even impossible, to diagnose. The only way possible indication is if the escape rhythm presents a QRS of a different pattern than the normal QRS during the atrial flutter.

2.5.8 Bradycardia owing to Artefacts

The recorder, especially if it is a tape recorder, may provoke false bradycardia by artefact. If, for any reason, the tape unwinds faster, it may result in a bradycardia which presents in addition the widening of all the recorded elements (QRS,P,T), enabling the correct interpretation.

2.5.9 Pauses Provoked by Artefacts

Actually, a pause or, better expressed, "a nontransitory recording" is much rarer with three leads. It is much more unlikely than with a single lead as the artefact has to be present on all three leads simultaneously, so we insist on having a Holter recording with at least three leads (see Sec. 3.4).

2.6 Cardiac Conduction Troubles

2.6.1 Sinoatrial Level and Sinoatrial Blocks

It is difficult, even impossible, to distinguish among a *sinus stop*, a *sinus pause*, and a *sinoatrial block*. We may speak of a sinoatrial block when we find a 2:1, 3:1, 3:2, etc., block on a tracing. If the pause without atrial activity is longer than two PP intervals, we prefer to speak of sinus pause or sinus stop.

It is advantageous to express this sinus pause or stop in terms of time, so it is important to measure its duration in relation to the PP interval. This is not always possible because the pause or the sinus stop may often be interrupted by an escape rhythm which is either supraventricular or ventricular. Before accepting the diagnosis of sinoatrial block, we must be sure that all the visible P waves are of sinus origin, and therefore they all must have the same morphology and appear in a rhythm that corresponds to the sinus rhythm. However, as we know that the sinus rhythm is never strictly regular, this makes the interpretation difficult. In the *differential diagnosis* we must definitely first consider blocked atrial premature beats.

These atrial premature beats usually fall in the repolarisation phase of the previous complex (ST-T segment) and as they modify this segment only slightly, they are very difficult to recognise. Their morphology must also be evaluated and it is only their chronology that allows us to make the correct diagnosis of ectopic origin (Fig. 2.18).

The sinus node has no expression on the electrocardiographic tracing, so the *sinoatrial block of the first degree* has no expression either. The *sinoatrial block of the second degree* may present the Wenckebach phenomenon and we may therefore distinguish between *type 1* and *type 2*. This is in analogy with the atrioventricular block. The type 1 in its usual form of 3:2 or 4:3 presents a PP interval which shortens to become shortest before the pause. This is due to the progressive lengthening of the conduction between the sinus node and the atria, and this lengthening is most significant at the beginning of the sequence. Since the sinus node atrial conduction recovers during the pause, the PP interval following the pause is slightly shorter than twice the PP distance. This shortening of the distance corresponds in principle to the duration of the sinoatrial conduction.

The *type 2 sinoatrial block* does not show the Wenckebach phenomenon. It presents a PP interval that is not progressively shortened, and the pause is twice that of the PP interval in sinus rhythm.

A *sinoatrial 2:1 block* provokes an important sinus bradycardia and should be suspected in the face of every important sinus bradycardia, that is, a heart rate that falls below 40 bpm (Fig. 2.19). To confirm or exclude this possibility, it is important to have a more prolonged and extended recording in order to follow the deceleration and acceleration of the cardiac rhythm. If we are witnessing a sinoatrial block, the deceleration and acceleration do not occur progressively, but follow the pattern of the block, as, for example, 3:2 or 4:3, or the frequency suddenly doubles with the disappearance of the block and the reappearance of 1:1 conduction.

A *third-degree sinoatrial block* presents in the form of an escape rhythm originating at different levels and replacing the cardiac rhythm.

An atrial mutism presents in the form of an escape rhythm with the absence of atrial activity. Diagnosis on the ECG Holter is impossible because we cannot preclude the possibility of hidden atrial activity in the previous QRS complex, which would inhibit the sinus activity.

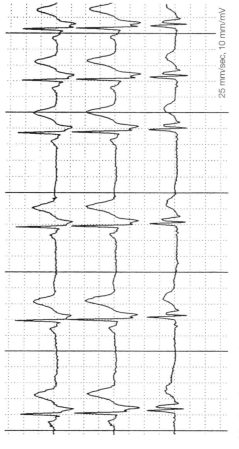

25 mm/sec, 10 mm/mV

Fig. 2.18 Sinus bradycardia of the first three complexes changes to sinus rhythm almost twice as fast. If we look carefully at the T waves from the bradycardic complexes, we see notching and an enhanced volume of the T wave (especially visible in the third lead). Therefore, we are not seeing a sinoatrial 2:1 block, but are rather in the presence of a bradycardia falsely induced by a blocked atrial bigeminism

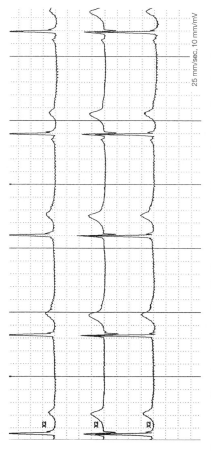

25 mm/sec, 10 mm/mV

Fig. 2.19 The first two complexes are of junctional origin. The third is also junctional, but on the ascending of the R wave, we see the added morphology of a P wave appearing progressively on the following complexes. This P wave is much more detached from the R wave, but we must note that it never conducts to the ventricle because the RR distance remains the same. Conclusion: isorhythmical dissociation between a junctional rhythm and a sinus bradycardia. The heart rate frequency of 38 bpm of the sinus activity is an indication that its vivacity must be checked

2.6.2 Atrioventricular Blocks

2.6.2.1 First-Degree Atrioventricular Block

A *first-degree atrioventricular block* manifests itself with the lengthening of the PR interval. As we have two or three bipolar thoracic leads at our disposal, the PR distance cannot be established with certitude because in these leads the beginning of the atrial activity may be isoelectrical. The PR interval shown on a Holter recording indicates the minimal distance from the atria to the ventricle but not necessarily the maximal distance. Therefore, even with this limitation, it is important to express the first-degree AV block in durationof the PR interval (in msec) (Fig. 2.20).

2.6.2.2 Second-Degree Atrioventricular Block

A *second-degree atrioventricular block* presents the same characteristics as those encountered on the clinical ECG; therefore the *type 1* presents a Wenckebach phenomenon with a progressive extension of the PR interval until the next P wave is not conducted. The extension is more marked at the beginning of the sequence and therefore the RR distance is narrowed, meaning that the RR distance is shorter before the pause. The *second-degree type 2 atrioventricular block* does not present this extension of the PR interval and the pause induced by the nonconductive P waves is exactly twice the duration of the RR interval.

2.6.2.3 Atrioventricular Block 2:1

A *2:1 atrioventricular block* must be expressed like this and cannot be quantified as type 1 or type 2 because the Wenckebach phenomenon cannot manifest itself. One has to follow the tracing to find the sequences that are 3:2 or 4:3, and it is only in these that the presence or absence of the Wenckebach phenomenon can be distinguished. If the Wenckebach phenomenon is found very often it situates the atrioventricular block at the nodal level. In the second-degree atrioventricular block, all P waves, and especially the nonconductive P waves, must be of sinus origin. The regularity of the sinus rhythm can be altered by a *ventriculophasia phenomenon*, which provokes a longer PP interval when there are no ventricular complexes between the P waves. This phenomenon may also exist in a complete atrioventricular block.

2.6.2.4 Second-Degree Advanced Atrioventricular Block

The *second-degree advanced atrioventricular block* (3:1, 4:1, 5:1, etc.) presents the same clinical characteristics as on a 12-lead electrocardiogram (Fig. 2.21).

2.6.2.5 Third-Degree Atrioventricular Block

The *third-degree or complete atrioventricular block* manifests itself in the same way as on the 12-lead electrocardiogram. The ventriculophasia phenomenon may render

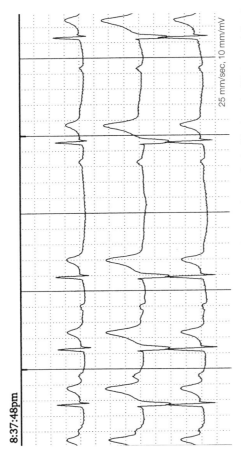

8:37:48pm

25 mm/sec, 10 mm/mV

Fig. 2.20 The first three complexes seem to be of sinus origin with a first-degree atrioventricular block and a PR interval that is slightly extended, from 0.30 to 0.40 sec for the third complex. We then see a pause which is twice the PP interval before the pause (1.76 × 1.84). The suggestion of sinoatrial block (2:1) seems to be plausible because we have no argument for any blocked premature atrial beat. On the complex following the pause, the PR interval is shortened to 0.28 sec. The last visible complex is also of sinus origin, with a PR interval of 0.40 sec. Conclusion: probable sinoatrial block 2:1, first-degree atrioventricular block with a Wenckebach phenomenon

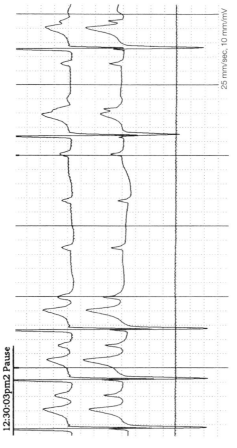

Fig. 2.21 We note a sinus rhythm of 84 bpm, transforming into an atrioventricular block. The three following P waves no longer conduct, and the fourth may seem to be conducted to the ventricular level, the next one is blocked, and a 2:1 atrioventricular block appears. Conclusion: advanced second-degree atrioventricular block responsible for a ventricular pause of 2.6 sec, 2:1 atrioventricular block

the P waves irregular. Unlike the clinical ECG which, at its maximum, records only some 12 sec, the ECG Holter may visualise captures from the sinus rhythm which indicate that the atrioventricular block is incomplete. Nevertheless, it is clinically important to use the term complete atrioventricular block if the captures are very isolated.

In a complete atrioventricular block we must look at the atrial activity, at its origin and its frequency. Moreover, since we are in a sinus activity it is important to determine its heart rate frequency and variability in order to be able to determine the sinus chronotropism so that we know what type of pacemaker should be implanted. If the atrial activity is an atrial fibrillation, it is important that we recognise this arrhythmia so that we can correctly indicate a full anticoagulation.

In the case of an atrial fibrillation with a complete atrioventricular block, the diagnosis is done with reference to a regular ventricular rhythm that remains slow. An intermittent irregularity may be difficult to interpret because it may be due to the presence of a capture of atrial activity from the atrial fibrillation, an extrasystoly from an escape rhythm, or a plurioriginality of the escape rhythm.

Capture from the atrial activity of the atrial fibrillation is the most common cause of intermittent irregularity. The regularity of the sinus rhythm in the presence of an atrioventricular block in addition to the ventriculophasia phenomenon may be stopped or modified by the presence of retrograde conduction (ventriculoatrial) of the escape rhythm. This may even be so if the escape rhythm is of ventricular origin. The atrioventricular block, even though it may be complete may allow a retrograde conduction. The atrial activity provoked by the retrograde conduction may modify the sinus activity or even inhibit it for a long period of time. This depends especially on the respective heart rate frequencies of the sinus activity and the retrograde atrial activity. This phenomenon may explain a symptomatology owing to the atrial contraction which occurs during the ventricular systoly. Moreover, this may be important for choosing the right type of permanent endocavitory stimulation and for programming the device correctly.

The irregularity of the escape rhythm may be due to captures from the sinus rhythm. In this case, a P wave must precede the captured complex. The capture may present a fusion phenomenon if the escape rhythm is of ventricular origin. In this case, the distance between the end of the preceding QRS escape rhythm and the end of the QRS of the capture with the fusion phenomenon is identical to the distance between the narrow QRS complexes of the escape rhythm.

Another origin of the irregularity of the escape rhythm is an extrasystoly, usually ventricular, and in this case the regularity of the *coupling* time may help us to arrive at the right diagnosis. The extrasystoly may have the very specific form of an echobeat, be linked to the escape rhythm, and, in principle, present all the morphology of a sinus rhythm, which means a bi- , tri- , or quadrigeminism, a doublet, or even a nonsustained tachycardia.

Another reason for the irregularity of an escape rhythm is the presence of two escape rhythms alternating with two different heart rate frequencies, and these usually present an incomplete dissociation with fusion phenomena.

2.6.2.6 Dynamic Evaluation of Cardiac Conduction Defects

It is always useful to evaluate the block during acceleration of the heart rate frequency. The block may disappear, may persist, or may worsen. Persistence or the worsening indicates an organic block, whereas the disappearance of the block during acceleration of the frequency is an indication of vagal origin. This is more evident with atrioventricular blocks.

2.6.3 Bundle Branch Blocks

It is impossible to determine the origin of the bundle branch blocks as one cannot determine intraventricular nonspecific conduction defects without a clinical 12-lead ECG with thoracic leads. Nevertheless, on a Holter recording it is possible to identify *phase 3 bundle branch blocks* (appearing during the acceleration period of the heart rate frequency) and *phase 4 bundle branch blocks* (appearing during the slowing of the heart rate frequency).

The appearance of the heart rate frequency of a phase 3 bundle branch block is not identical to its disappearance frequency. Both frequencies must be noted because they may evolve into a *permanent bundle branch block* or potentially into a complete atrioventricular block. The *phase 4 bundle branch block* is much less common. The differential diagnosis with an escape ventricular rhythm is not easy, but its presence signifies the probability of progression to a complete atrioventricular block, which should not be underestimated.

2.6.4 Preexcitation

Preexcitation with a difficult WPW morphology is not easily diagnosed on a Holter recording. The PR interval does not have the same value as the PR interval on a clinical ECG because the beginning of the P wave may be hidden in the isoelectric signal of the Holter leads.

The preexcitation itself (the delta wave) has no axial expression and the beginning of the R wave may not be easy to distinguish. Nevertheless, a preexcitation may disappear with the acceleration of the heart rate frequency or alternatively may appear in the slow heart rate frequencies when the nodo-Hisian conduction pathway is slowed by the vagal nerve, wherefore the conduction preferentially takes place over the aberrant pathway (as, e.g., the Kent bundle).

The orthodromic tachycardias of the WPW syndrome present a P wave close to the previous QRS complex (the RP distance is shorter than the PR distance). The antidromic tachycardias are much less common and present quite an unusually wide QRS.

2.7 ST Segment Analysis

2.7.1 Generalities

The ST segment, by definition, goes from the end of the QRS (usually the end of the S waves) to the beginning of the T wave. The end of the S wave is also called the *J point*. This segment corresponds to phase 2 of the action potential, also called *the plateau*. It is quite easy to see where the S wave and the J point are at the end of the ventricular complex, but it is quite often difficult to locate the beginning of the T wave.

The ST segment is the expression of a precarious equilibrium and is recorded normally as an isoelectric line. The equilibrium can be altered easily and there are many conditions, some of them *physiological* and others *pathological* that produce an ST segment change, either an *ascent* or a *descent*. The former are more common than the latter. The physiological conditions are usually the ones that relate to the autonomous innervations (as, e.g., the change of position when one goes from a sitting up, to a lying down, or a standing position or hyperventilation, and so on). In terms of pathological origin, the most important things to consider are, for example, ischemia, ventricular hypertrophy, intraventricular conduction defect, pericarditis, ionic disorder, and the effects of different medications.

The reproducibility, the specificity, and the sensibility of an ST segment recording and the determination of the isoelectric level are not very good and it will take time to improve them. Therefore, the analyses of the ST segment on a Holter recording take time to be interpretable, even though, N. J. Holter showed the presence of a myocardiac ischemia in his first publication.

For these reasons, the use of the ECG Holter to record modifications of the ST segment has been challenged. It took time to prove that the recorders modulated by amplitude (*AM recorder*) are as trustworthy in the recording of deep frequencies as are the frequency-modulated recorders (*FM recorders*).

Currently, both these systems are at our disposal for general clinical practice; the AM recorder has recently been improved for the correct recording of the slow frequencies and now reproduces the ST segment as well as the FM recorder. Both systems interact with the backward electricity, which is the cause of many artefacts.

Recently, new recorders with real time analyses have been introduced. There is an analytic system is at one's disposal and the detection and classification parameters can be modified by the clinical reader. Nevertheless, visual control is always important for the doctor to evaluate the quantitative and the qualitative presence of these ST segment modifications.

2.7.2 Myocardial Ischemia

Myocardial ischemia can be diagnosed in the presence of electrocardiographic changes, including a *descent of the ST segment* which is either *descending* or *horizontal*, definitively more than 0.1 mV, and appearing gradually for at least 1 min and disappearing for at least the same length of time before eventually reappearing again. Each episode of transient ischemia must be separated by a period of at least 1 min during which the ST segment again becomes isoelectric. Some authors prefer a normal period that is almost 5 min long, because the end of the first episode and the beginning of the second often last more than 1 min. Taking account of this definition, we see that there are no limits on the *duration of the transient ischemic episode*. It nevertheless seems logical that an ischemia may hardly last more than 30 min (which is the same length of time as the clinical definition of *angor pectoris*). The automatic reading of ST segment deviation by superimposition must be verified on the classical printed ECG Holter that is produced manually by the operator. The appearance and the disappearance of the ST segment must be seen by a human eye (Figs. 2.22 and 2.23).

To look at the ST segment descent one must focus on 60 or 80 msec following the J point. In some circumstances *it is advisable not to diagnose myocardial ischemia*:

- In the presence of a rhythm that is not a sinus rhythm and especially in atrial fibrillation or flutter.
- In the presence on the clinical 12-lead electrocardiogram of a ventricular left hypertrophy, a bundle branch block (especially if it is the left bundle branch block), a nonspecific intraventricular conduction defect with a widened QRS of more than 0.10 sec, or preexcitation.
- In association with some medication, in particular drugs such as digoxine, amiodarone, flecainide, antidepressive drugs, and diuretics.
- In the presence of a very serious ionic disorder.

To optimise diagnostic precision, one must be very careful when placing electrodes, the skin must be carefully prepared (to diminish impedance), and one must choose the electrode position which simulates a normal 12-lead ECG lead derivation V5 and V1; one must be able to recognise a preponderant R wave that is over 10 mm in size. To do so and to be able to find the same size V5 and V1 position with that kind of a wave, one must place the electrodes on the bones to diminish the muscular potential and be very careful in fixing the cables because movement can affect the isoelectric line.

We are interested in performing a long-duration ST segment recording especially in three categories of patient :

- The first population is made up of patients with known coronary artery disease who present a symptomatic *angina pectoris*. In this population, we find in addition to the ST segment changes at the moment of the pain, asymptomatic ST segment changes which are quite obvious and pathognomonic, and indicate the existence of silent ischemia. It appears that the presence of silent ischemia worsens the prognosis in this population.
- The second population includes patients with a probable coronary artery disease (uncertain) who do not present with clinical pain but where we find the kind of

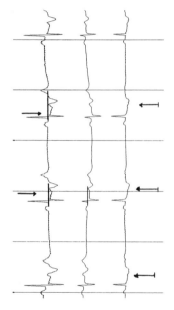

Fig. 2.22 The false sinus bradycardia is caused by a blocked atrial bigeminism (the lower arrows), which then provokes a myocardial ischemia. It shows essentially in the third lead with an ST segment descent (top arrows with visualisation of the isoelectric level). The patient was asymptomatic as this recording was made during the night. Conclusion: atrial blocked bigeminism, provoking a silent myocardial ischemia with ST segment descent

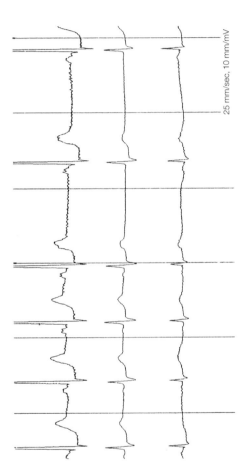

25 mm/sec, 10 mm/mV

Fig. 2.23 Normal sinus rhythm of 70 bpm is interrupted by a premature atrial beat which remains blocked, and the heart rate falls to 40 bpm. The same phenomenon appears once more. There is an important difference in the ST segment morphology when the premature atrial blocked phenomenon is present and when it is not. We also note a deep ST segment descent which is horizontal in the first lead, indicating a silent asymptomatic myocardial ischemia. This phenomenon lasts for 10 min on the recording

ST segment changes that correspond to myocardial ischemia. In these cases a diagnosis of the silent myocardial ischemia is very likely.

- The third population, patients without coronary artery disease and without any symptomatology during the recording, speaks to the discovery of coronary artery disease in an asymptomatic patient with a seemingly healthy heart, so it is very important to eliminate any factor that might influence the ST segment before writing a diagnosis of silent myocardial ischemia. In case of any doubt, another examination to detect myocardial ischemia as, for example, either a stress test, including nuclear cardiology testing, or magnetic resonance imaging (MRI) testing should be considered.

Large variations in the ST segment changes from one recording to another must also be considered, especially if we want to show the efficiency of a medical treatment or the positive effect of an invasive procedure. Even though the ST segment horizontal descent is the sign most commonly diagnosed in the presence of myocardial ischemia, an ST segment ascent can also be a sign of transmural ischemia, which may be provoked by an important proximal coronary stenosis or in the presence of a Prinzmetal angina.

From recent American and world guidelines there is no *class I indication* (meaning either very strong evidence or a general consensus as to the usefulness or efficiency of this technique) for a 24-hr Holter recording for myocardial ischemia. There is a *class II indication* (meaning that there is not a consensus but dominant opinion favours its use). This class II indication can either be a *class Ia* where the opinion is in favour of use, as is essentially the case in Prinzmetal angina, or it may be a *class Ib*, where usefulness is much less evident, as in the case of patients with atypical or typical chest pain who are not able to perform a stress test and do present an indication for surgery. There are no *class III indications*, as, for example, to evaluate the initial chest pains in patients who can perform a stress test. There is also no indication for routine detection in asymptomatic patients.

The recommendationsfor detection of myocardial ischemia speak in favour of stress tests because whatever the mode of stress, this test is performed with a full 12-lead recording; there are many fewer artefacts and these can be corrected for during the test. It is also important to remember that the Holter recording is read afterwards, and therefore the patient, if the diagnosis is correct, suffers from ischemia without any opportunity for the doctor to treat him at the time of the manifestation.

2.8 ECG Holter and Pacemakers

2.8.1 Generalities

2.8.1.1 Current Programming

During the last 10 years, pacemakers have benefited from remarkable technical development. To interpret the ECG Holter correctly, it is important to know the exact type of the pacemaker (PM), and the way it was programmed, as well as the mode of stimulation at the moment of the ECG recording and all of the activated algorithms.

Every patient with a PM, has a card, either European or from the country of implantation, which should list all the characteristics of the PM, including the current programmed parameters. The technician who fixes the Holter recording device must copy all the data which are indispensable for a correct interpretation:

- The PM type
- The stimulation mode (AAI, VVI, DDD, VDD, DVI, DDI)
- Stimulation polarity (unipolar or bipolar)
- The presence or absence of rate responsiveness (R)
- The minimal and maximal heart rate frequency
- The different algorithms that are activated at the moment of the recording.

2.8.1.2 Stimulation Mode

The PM may stimulate only at the atrial level (*AAI*), only at the ventricular level (*VVI*), or at both levels (*DDD, DDI*). This stimulation mode can be programmed and may even automatically change in the presence of different algorithms during the recording.

The *first letter* in the three-letter code indicates the *stimulation cavity* (Atrial, Ventricular, Double cavity), the *second letter* the cavity where the *sensing* is done, and the *third letter* how the sensing is treated: *I* meaning that the PM is inhibited after the sensing, *T* meaning the sensing triggers stimulation, and *D* meaning that at the ventricular level the PM is inhibited but at the same time, the sensing at the atrial level will provoke a stimulation at the ventricular level (*VAT*).

2.8.1.3 Stimulation on Demand

The actual stimulation is usually *on demand*, which means that the PM is activated (provokes the spike) only after a duration which is given by its programmed stimulation frequency (expressed in milliseconds, which gives the stimulation period) following either the last spontaneous complex sensed or the last triggered complex. Therefore, a PM programmed at 60 bpm presents a stimulation period of 1000 ms.

2.8.1.4 Stimulation Polarity

Possibly *unipolar*, stimulation takes place between one of the leads that is in the cavity being stimulated (atria or ventricle) and the metallic part of the PM device itself. The unipolar stimulation (unipolar spikes) is usually quite visible on a Holter tracing.

Bipolar stimulation is actually between the two electrodes on the lead which is present in its respective cardiac cavity. The bipolar spikes are very often barely visible on the tracing. We must remember that the stimulation may be unipolar in one cavity, often the ventricle, and bipolar in the other cavity (atria). This allows us to distinguish the atrial spike from the ventricular spike more easily.

2.8.1.5 Stimulation Trigger

The triggering of the PM (spike) is an electrical descent of a very short duration (usually 0.5 ms), and this is the reason for its imperceptibility on the tracing. On some Holter recording devices there is a *PM option*, which is activated on the recording device; every time it recognises a spike it provokes an artificial deflection on the recording which is easy to diagnose. The advantage is having well-drawn spikes on the tracing. Unfortunately, this type of assistance is not 100% efficient because nothing can mimic a spike as well as an artefact; if one activates this option, it is the computer analysis that decides what should be kept on the tracing as a spike and there is no possible visual control. It is much more difficult to distinguish a spike from an artefact if the recorder has artificially and uniformly designed spikes on the tracing. On a usual tracing without the PM option, even though the spikes are not well represented, they may actually be much easier to distinguish from false artificial spikes because it is the human eye that makes the decision, and the human brain remains superior to the computer in arriving at a correct diagnosis.

2.8.1.6 Rate Responsiveness of Stimulation

The *rate responsiveness may be programmed* (*R* as the fourth letter) to accelerate the heart rate frequency from the *minimal* to the *maximal* stimulation frequency (both being programmable)(Fig. 2.24).

2.8.1.7 Hysteresis

The presence of a programmable *hysteresis* extends the time before the appearance of the next stimulation (meaning the stimulation period from the last spontaneous complex) by comparing the times (stimulation period) between two successive stimulations.

2.8.1.8 Minimal Stimulation Frequency

Programmed in the DDD PM, this determines the frequency at which the DDD PM starts to stimulate at the atrial level. The ventricles are only stimulated if the atrioventricular spontaneous conduction is absent or too prolonged (longer than the programmed atrioventricular stimulation time).

2.8.1.9 Maximal Stimulation Frequency

The *maximal stimulation* frequency (programmed) is that frequency that may not be overridden by the ventricular stimulation following the sensing of the spontaneous atrial activity (VAT). The limit on this maximal frequency is not usually abrupt,

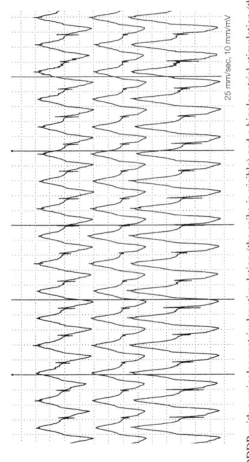

25 mm/sec, 10 mm/mV

Fig. 2.24 We note a PM DDDR with a unipolar ventricular stimulation (the spike is visible) and a bipolar atrial stimulation (the spike is less visible); it is more noticeable in the first lead at the top of the T wave. As the atrial stimulation is also accelerated we must be in a rate responsive mode. This rate goes up to 160 bpm on both the atrial and the ventricular levels; it is very important to assess the patient's activity during this moment of the recording, as well as to know the patient's age to be sure that such a rate responsive high rate is advisable

but rather occurs with a progressive artificial Wenckebach type of atrioventricular blockage (Fig. 2.25).

2.8.1.10 Algorithms

The activated presence of different *algorithms* may modify the ECG Holter:

(a) The *stimulation mode commutation* algorithm commutes the stimulation mode from a DDD PM (or DDD-R PM) to a VVI or VVIR stimulation, when a spontaneous atrial tachyarrhythmia occurs (atrial fibrillation or flutter) and this stops the ventricular stimulation from following the ectopic atrial activity, which is then too fast. Once the rhythm reverts to normal sinus rhythm and is correctly recognised by the device, the PM automatically commutes back to the DDD (or DDD-R) stimulation.

(b) The *safety ventricular pacing* algorithm once programmed is activated when sensing at the ventricular level is uncertain following an atrial spike and provokes a ventricular stimulation in a shortened atrioventricular interval (100–120 ms) (Fig. 2.26). If the uncertain sensing is a true ventricular complex, the ventricular spike provoked by the algorithm is in a complete refractory ventricular period which is absolute owing to the shortening of the atrioventricular interval. If the spike is provoked by the usual atrioventricular interval as it was programmed, the ventricular spike could fall in a vulnerable ventricular phase. If the uncertain sensing is not a ventricular complex, the spike provokes ventricular capture much sooner after the atrial spike and therefore does not represent any rhythmic risk.

(c) Other algorithms may be present and may modify the recording, as, for instance: (i) the algorithm that determines the stimulation threshold and the automatic enhancement or decrease of the stimulation energy; (ii) the algorithm that looks for spontaneous atrioventricular conduction by automatically increasing the atrioventricular programmed interval.

2.8.1.11 Counting System

Most current PMs benefit from a *counting system* of stimulated and spontaneous complexes. This system also records the heart rate frequency of both and indicates the presence of fast spontaneous complexes, both from the atria and the ventricle. These analyses can only be seen at the moment of the PM's control. These events are demonstrated by histograms, usually expressed in percentages and they give a lot of useful information on the presence or absence of arrhythmia and on the proper or incorrect functioning of the PM. Nevertheless, whereas for the time being these systems cannot replace the ECG Holter, they do provide useful additional information. Very often, the much cruder database from the interrogation of a PM device leads to an indication to perform a full 24-hr (or 48-hr) Holter assessment which has much more condensed information and much greater accuracy.

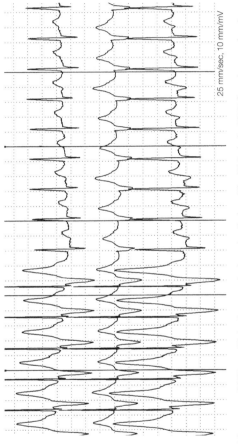

Fig. 2.25 DDD PM, maximal heart rate 130 bpm. Unipolar ventricular stimulation. The PM via its VAT function reaches its maximal frequency of 130 bpm. It then stops the stimulation abruptly because the patient presents an underlying spontaneous rhythm of 150 bpm

25 mm/sec, 10 mm/mV

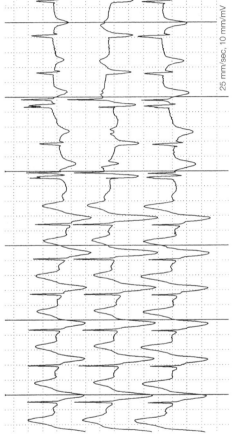

25 mm/sec, 10 mm/mV

Fig. 2.26 DDDR PM. Owing to its VAT, the PM follows the accelerated sinus rhythm which is at first around 125 bpm and then accelerates to 130 bpm. Because of an extended programmed refractory period (PVARP), the PM does not capture the last spontaneous P wave and starts to stimulate according to its R programmed function, which at this point is around 80 bpm. The atrial spike falls into the spontaneous QRS (pseudo-pseudofusion), so the safety ventricular stimulation algorithm is activated. As a consequence, we see that the ventricular spike is at a distance of 0.08 from the atrial spike (especially visible in the first lead). The next complex is not sensed and the PM provokes a new pseudo-pseudofusion, but this time without the ventricular stimulation safety algorithm (the atrial spike was too late for the spontaneous ventricular complex). We then see three spontaneous complexes whose P waves are hidden in the T waves and thus are not sensed because of the refractory period. On the other hand, the ventricular complexes are well sensed. Profound negative T waves in the spontaneous complexes are probably due to the Chatterjee phenomenon

We must not forget that the counting devices present in the different PMs are endocavitary recordings of the atrial or ventricular potentials, and not a recording taken from the body surface.

2.8.1.12 Fusion

A *fusion* is an activation created simultaneously by the PM spike and the spontaneous activity. Even though fusions exist at the atrial level (*P wave fusion*), we usually speak of *ventricular fusions*. The fusion ventricular complex is narrowly preceded by the spike, and its aspect is more or less different from the ventricular complex which is only stimulated and is less wide. A *pseudofusion* is a ventricular complex in which the spike occurred too late in the QRS to be able to activate it even for a very small portion of the ventricle, and therefore the QRS morphology is only slightly modified by the spike, which would have a spontaneous complex aspect if the latter were not added to it (Fig. 2.27). A *pseudo pseudofusion ventricular* is identical to a pseudofusion but the spike is of atrial origin.

2.8.2 Interpretation of Pacemaker Function

The correct interpretation of the ECG Holter recording in a PM patient must at least answer three main questions: *Is there a failure to pace, a failure to capture, or a failure to sense?*

2.8.2.1 Failure to Pace

A spike is missing in the fixed stimulation period, following the last stimulated complex or spontaneous complex and the consequence is a pause that is longer than the programmed stimulation period but which keeps the period's multiplicity duration. The cause of the failure-to-pace defect is an electronic one in the genesis of the PM's stimulus which nowadays is actually a rare and unusual fault. A pause in the absence of a spike is often provoked by a failure to sense (see Sec. 2.8.2.3).

2.8.2.2 Failure to Capture

Failure to capture is manifested by a spike which is not followed by a capture response (falling in a period out of the refractory period for the cavity concerned). This means that either the spike energy is insufficient to stimulate or that the lead has lost contact with the cavity wall where the stimulation should take place. Even in an intermittent form, this failure to capture is a very serious complication because it means that we cannot be certain that the stimulation takes place in all circumstances.

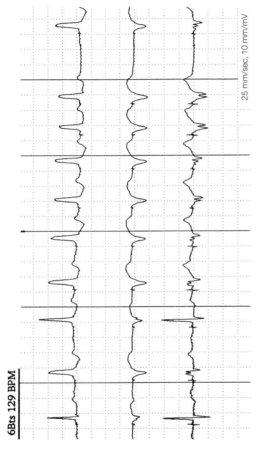

Fig. 2.27 DDD PM, bipolar stimulation. The first complex is a sinus complex with a relatively long PR interval and the ventricular spike is released without activating the ventricle (pseudofusion). We then see an atrial premature beat which leads to the ventricle via the PM (VAT). The next complex is similar to the first one and is again of sinus origin. This time the ventricular spike modifies the QRS morphology, which is especially visible if one compares it to the first complex by suppressing the S wave (in the first lead) and modifying the global morphology in the second lead. We are then in the presence of a fusion. We then see an atrial tachycardia of six QRS transmitted to the PM via the ventricular level. The last two complexes of the tachycardia are fully activated by the ventricular spike. Therefore, we can say that for the previous complexes a spontaneous conduction was present. This means that even without a PM, this atrial tachycardia would trigger the ventricle (but perhaps not in the last two complexes). Following the cessation of the tachycardia we see a pause terminated by an atrial and a ventricular stimulation. The atrial capture is not seen clearly. The ventricular complex presents fusion signs because of its morphology and thus confirms the atrial capture

2.8.2.3 Failure to Sense

To stimulate on demand, the PM must sense spontaneous activity in each cavity. The failure to sense may manifest itself in two forms:

(a) The PM cannot sense the electrical potential of the spontaneous activity, and in this case the spike is triggered without taking account of the spontaneous activity. This results in a fixed triggering (*undersensing*).

(b) The PM senses an inadequate cardiac electrical potential (e.g., the T wave) or an extracardiac potential (e.g., a potential provoked by the contraction of peripheral muscles), considers it to be a spontaneous activity in the cardiac cavity concerned, and recycles itself from the false supernumerous sensing (*oversensing*). In this case, it may result in a pause without any cardiac activity as long as the extracardiac potential lasts. The pause is not a multiple of the stimulation period. In case of muscular potential, the tracing is often full of parasites provoked by the potential itself. There may be other sources for this oversensing, and these must be noted in the patient's logbook, and addressed during the clinical consilium following the Holter recording. The patient must be asked if he or she was using any electrical devices or was in a particular electrical environment at the moment of the manifestation.

These two failure-to-sense types may also modify the function of triggering the ventricular stimulation upon the atrial sensing (VAT). In the first case, when the PM does not recognise the activity potential, it may result in the absence of a ventricular stimulation, which may lead to a decrease in the ventricular heart rate if the defect is intermittent or to a brutal ventricular stimulation fall to the minimum programmed if the defect maintains itself for an extended period. The rate responsiveness of the stimulation (DDDR) determines the frequency of the ventricular stimulation if it is programmed (Fig. 2.28).

In the second case of failure to sense, in the presence of oversensing, the PM presents a particular defect: *cross talk of DDD PMs*. In this case, the PM senses the electrical potential of the atrial stimulus (spike) at the ventricular level and as a consequence there is no true ventricular spike leading to a ventricular pause. To prevent this defect, the PM presents a *blanking period* following the atrial spike whose duration is programmable and which should normally prevent the cross talk. The phenomenon of the *electrical polarisation* provoked by the atrial spike whose energy is increased may prolong the electric potential further than the blanking period, and provoke cross talk nevertheless.

2.8.3 Pacemaker Tracings and Spontaneous Rhythms

The ECG Holter *interpretation* system must also interpret and understand the characteristics of normal spontaneous complexes and rhythms.

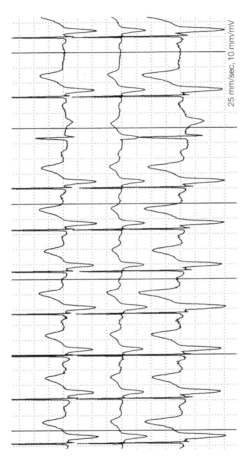

25 mm/sec, 10 mm/mV

Fig. 2.28 DDDR PM. The PM follows the sinus rhythm via VAT by stimulating the ventricles with a heart rate frequency of 110 bpm. The eighth P wave is not sensed and the ventricular spike is missing. The next two P waves are once more correctly sensed and provoke ventricular stimulation. Conclusion: intermittent sensing defect at the atrial level

2.8.3.1 Spontaneous Activity at the Atrial Level

The *spontaneous activity* at the atrial level is very important in determining the basic rhythm. It can be of sinus origin with spontaneous P waves showing a sinus appearance. In this case, we must note the maximal and minimal heart rate in this rhythm, which, in relation to the physical activity during the recording, is a reflection of the *sinus chronotropism* (Fig. 2.29).

The spontaneous atrioventricular conduction state must also be noted:

(a) It can be absent or longer than the programmed atrioventricular interval, and in this case, each P wave is followed by a ventricular spike from a DDD PM (VAT).
(b) It is possible but not fast enough and from time to time we find fusion complexes which may also be associated with pseudofusion complexes. This depends on the ratio between the duration of the spontaneous atrioventricular conduction and the programmed atrioventricular interval. This may be modified by the heart rate frequency because the spontaneous conduction may not be able to adapt to the heart rate acceleration; on the other hand, the atrioventricular interval may be programmed dynamically, which means that this interval shortens with the acceleration of the heart rate.

The *spontaneous* conduction must be recognised and interpreted correctly because it is symmetrical without a left bundle branch block, and this means hemodynamical advantages. For this reason, it is useful to know when spontaneous atrioventricular conduction occurs so that we can have optimal programming of the PM device. There is also an algorithm which looks for spontaneous atrioventricular conduction by automatically increasing the atrioventricular interval. The atrioventricular conduction dysfunctions can be intermittent, and in this case a sinus rhythm leading to the ventricles may be present.

The sinus rhythm at the atrial level may be interrupted by *atrial fibrillation or flutter*. The ventricular stimulation follows the atrial activity to its programmed maximal frequency (DDD PM). The atrial fibrillation presents fibrillation Fwaves of a very different electrical potential, which may vary from beat to beat, so atrial sensing may be very irregular or not even there at all. Hence, it provokes an atrial stimulation of minimal frequency without any atrial capture, followed by a ventricular stimulation which depends on the spontaneous atrioventricular conduction of the atrial fibrillation. In case of a fast atrial sense, the ventricles may follow to the maximal stimulation frequency programmed on the device.

The *commutation mode's algorithm* automatically changes the DDD stimulation to VVI or from DDDR to VVIR and once the arrhythmia stops, it commutes from VVI to DDD stimulation or from VVIR to DDDR. Atrial fibrillation or flutter can totally replace the sinus rhythm and in this case the atria cannot be stimulated. Even in the presence of the VVI PM, the atrial flutter or fibrillation must be noted because its presence is an indication for anticoagulant treatment.

Premature atrial beats may occur, and in this case it is useful to know whether their conduction to the ventricle is mediated only by the PM or if they may be

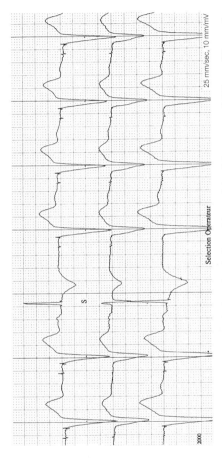

Fig. 2.29 DDD PM, bipolar stimulation. Atrial and ventricular stimulation with a minimal heart rate of 60 bpm. We see the appearance of a spontaneous complex preceded by a P wave with a sinus morphology. The sinus complex is detected clearly; very often there is a programmable difference in the atrioventricular interval, depending on whether we are in the presence of a stimulated interval (i.e., an interval between the atrial and the ventricular spikes) or in a sensed interval (i.e., an interval between the sensed P wave and the ventricular spike). The deep negative T waves are an expression of the Chatterjee phenomenon

conducted spontaneously. Furthermore, when in the presence of an atrial tachycardia, it is very important to know whether it is transmitted to the ventricle mediated by the PM or if it is maintained spontaneously.

2.8.3.2 Spontaneous Activity at the Ventricular Level

The *spontaneous activity at the ventricular level* may manifest itself by premature ventricular beats, by ventricular tachycardia, and eventually by an accelerated idioventricular rhythm (AIVR). As we do not know what the spontaneous ventricular complex looks like, it is possible that not every wide QRS spontaneous complex is of ventricular origin. It would be useful at this point to have the reading of a 12-lead electrocardiogram, especially before the implantation of the PM device to adequately determine the complex. It is also useful to find a spontaneous supraventricular complex in the tracing in order to see the morphology of each QRS.

When we observe ventricular premature beats, it is useful to know whether they appear only in the presence of the pace rhythm, if they occur in spontaneous rhythm, or if they seem not to be connected with any of the rhythms. The same characterisation should take place in the case of ventricular tachycardia. In the presence of all ventricular arrhythmias, it is very important to look at the ventricular sensing and specifically search for a spike in the arrhythmia, which indicates a failure to sense. In theory, a ventricular premature beat perpendicular to the axis formed by the bipolar sensing of the electrodes may present a potential which is merely nil and so may not be sensed by the device.

To be able to determine spontaneous atrioventricular conduction, it is necessary to identify the completely paced ventricular complex, which usually represents the widest complex. We often find it at the limiting heart rate frequencies, comparing all the paced complexes; we might also recognise the fusion phenomenon, which means that there is spontaneous atrioventricular conduction.

2.8.3.3 Pacemaker Syndrome

The *PM syndrome* manifests itself after the implantation of a pacemaker (usually VVI or VVIR) on clinical presentation of palpitations associated with aches, vertigo, and even loss of consciousness. On the ECG, we find that the syndrome appears when a spontaneous rhythm is replaced by a stimulated rhythm (VVI or VVIR) which, by retrograde conduction, makes retrograde P waves appear in the middle of the ventricular systoly. The slight decrease in the cardiac output, already provoked by the stimulated rhythm (VVI), is enhanced by the atrial contractions occurring against closed atrioventricular valves. The increase in the pressure in the pulmonary veins stimulates the baroreceptors and provokes a reflex hypotension. The clinical presentation of a PM syndrome is very individual and retrograde P waves may exist without any such clinical manifestation.

2.8.3.4 Electronic Reentrant Tachycardia

A *PM-mediated tachycardia* may appear during DDD stimulation when a retrograde P wave is sensed at the atrial level of the PM and provokes a ventricular stimulation (VAT) which once more causes a retrograde P wave that stimulates a tachycardia by repetition. The frequency of this tachycardia cannot be more than the maximal programmed stimulated frequency.

2.8.4 Summary of the Different Stimulation Modes on the ECG Holter

1. AAI/AAIR stimulation is very rarely used because it necessitates a normal atrioventricular conduction (even in the future). The atrial capture is not often recognisable, and in this case the AV conduction with ventricular response may be there as a witness of the atrial capture, especially during acceleration (AAIR). The spontaneous atrioventricular conduction should be identified and its lengthening with acceleration noted, as it could reflect rate responsiveness acceleration, which is not justified clinically.

2. VVI/VVIR stimulation is the oldest stimulation but it is still used frequently, especially for patients with permanent or predominant atrial fibrillation. The regularities of the ventricular contractions may mask the atrial fibrillation, but when the latter is present, there is a strict injunction to continue anticoagulant therapy.

3. DDD/DDDR stimulation includes AAI stimulation with VVI stimulation and the VAT function. Nowadays, it is quite predominant programming, although it is rather complex owing to the presence of different algorithms.

The acceleration of the ventricular stimulation frequency may follow spontaneous atrial activity (VAT), in which case there is no atrial spike, or it may occur with the frequency responsiveness, in which case, there is an atrial spike. The two ways of acceleration may occur concomitantly. The ECG Holter may provide important information on optimising the programming of the device.

The presence of intermittent atrial arrhythmia may enhance functioning of DDD PM, because the VAT function may accelerate the ventricular stimulation without any real hemodynamical cause. The various commutation mode algorithms try to avoid these unnecessary accelerations, which are perceived clinically as palpitations (see Secs. 2.8.1.10 and 2.8.3.1). The DDD PM can present cross talk (see Sec. 2.8.2.3) and provoke a PM-mediated tachycardia (see Sec. 2.8.3.4).

4. VDD/VDDR stimulation looks quite similar to the VAT function of the DDD PM but there is no atrial stimulation. The atria are used for sensing, which is done through floating leads. In the case of a sensing defect or the appearance of atrial fibrillation, some PMs may switch into VVI and others into VVIR.

5. DVI/DVIR is a two-level stimulation, on demand on the ventricular level (VVI) but fixed (AOO) at the atrial level. The VAT function is not present. The ventricular stimulation can only accelerate with the rate responsiveness (R).

6. DDI/DDIR shows a two-level stimulation (AAI and VVI) but without a VAT function, meaning without a ventricular stimulation that depends on the atrial sensing.

2.8.5 *Example of a Holter ECG Report Pacemaker Patient*

At the top of the report, we list the PM characteristics:

- Type
- Stimulation mode
- Stimulation frequency
- Stimulation polarity
- Presence or absence of rate responsiveness
- Programmed atrioventricular delay

Then:

- Presence of spontaneous rhythm and its form at the atrial and ventricular level
- Sinus chronotropism in the DDD or VDD pacemakers
- The atrioventricular conduction state
- The presence and maximal heart rate mediated by the VAT stimulation (for DDD and VDD pacemakers)
- The maximal frequency during rate responsiveness

Then

- The basic pacemaker functions (at the ventricular and/or atrial level) which indicate the presence or absence of: (i) failure to pace, (ii) failure to capture, (iii) undersensing and oversensing.

Only after all of the above have been accounted for should one note the presence of arrhythmias at the atrial and/or ventricular level and their relationship to the stimulation. The presence of retrograde P waves, of PM-mediated tachycardia, and of different algorithms should then be noted. Finally, one should study the description of the tracing recorded during the clinically described symptoms.

Chapter 3
Presenting ECG Holter Data

Evaluating the Recording, Display Counting, Statistics, and Graphic Expression of the Sensed and Interpreted Information

3.1 Frequency Trend

The *frequency trend* expresses the nycthemeral profile of the 24-hr period. The average frequency indicates the acceleration during daily activities and the slowing down during sleep, and in this way reflects the neurohormonal activity. The trend modifications, either by flattening (e.g., in diabetic neuropathy) or by enhancement (e.g., in neurovegetative dystonia) can lead to the correct diagnosis of a specific pathology (Fig. 3.1).

3.2 Hourly Expressions

The *hourly expressions* of the heart rate frequency expressed in average, minimal, and maximal frequency add a great deal to the information, particularly to the frequency trend (Fig. 3.2).

The monitored values must be associated with the activities in order to judge the adjustment or nonadjustment of the physical form. A cardiac frequency accelerated in all hourly recordings without an adequate corresponding physical activity suggests anaemia, hyperthyroidism, etc. Inadequate acceleration of the heart rate during the day is an indication of a physical inaptitude or a subclinical cardiac insufficiency.

On the other hand, if a bradycardia predominates even though the patient presents physical activity, once we have ruled out hypothyroidism, we must consider that the sinus function may not be optimal (dyschronotropism) or that the patient takes bradycardiac medication, such as a beta blocker. One must not forget that eye drops, which the patient sometimes forgets to mention in the clinical history, have beta-blocking agents.

J. Adamec, R. Adamec, *ECG Holter*, DOI: 10.1007/978-0-387-78187-7_3,
© Springer Science+Business Media, LLC 2008

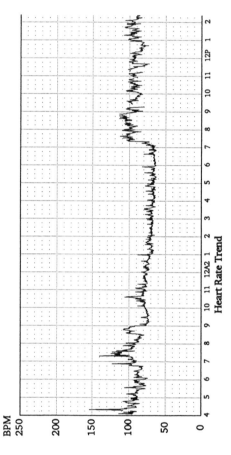

Fig. 3.1 The heart rate frequency trend presents a curve which may be considered as normal, the lowest heart rate frequencies being around 60 bpm at night and the daytime heart rate acceleration being in accordance with the physical activity

HOUR ENDG	TOTAL BEATS	--HEART RATE--			----VENTRICULAR ECTOPICS---				
		MIN	MAX	AVG	TOTAL	/1000	BIGEM	PAIR	RonT
1pm	4967	73	97	88	176	35		2	
2	5688	86	107	94	296	52		32	
3	5201	80	102	87	274	53	3	12	
4	4786	77	96	83	188	39	5	8	
5	4909	76	95	83	167	34		2	
6	4783	73	92	81	214	45		2	
7	4751	72	89	80	190	40		8	
8	4792	74	95	81	122	25		2	
9	5021	74	96	85	234	47	6	12	
10	4774	75	97	83	279	58	3	10	
11	4756	70	85	79	227	48		8	
12am2	4765	73	86	79	105	22	4	8	
1am2	4610	71	86	77	37	8			
2	4655	72	83	78	39	8		2	
3	4607	70	98	77	59	13		2	
4	4414	72	83	74	96	22		4	
5	4430	70	82	74	88	20	6	6	
6	4636	70	86	77	37	8			
7	4931	71	100	82	104	21		6	
8	4799	74	90	80	57	12			
9	5314	77	107	92	165	31	3	4	
10	6205	86	121	103	351	57		20	
11	5183	76	107	85	137	26		4	
1157am	4459	73	89	77	70	16		4	

Fig. 3.2 Hourly monitoring of the heart rate frequencies. We also see the repartition of the premature ventricular beats. The minimal heart rate frequency never goes below 70 bpm. There is evidence of numerous premature ventricular beats, essentially during the day, which diminish in frequency by more than half during night and reappear quite strongly after the patient wakes up. Therefore, we are in the presence of catecholinergic ventricular premature beats and should look for a cardiac insufficiency

3.3 Histograms

The various *histograms* reflect the repartition in time of the premature beats and tachycardias in a more illustrative way. Daytime repartition suggests a catecholamine role and night time repartition is an indication of a vagal role, whereas the presence of premature beats without repartition evokes a toxic (e.g., digitalis) or an organic effect.

3.4 Electrocardiographic Transcription

The electrocardiographic transcription of different recordings necessitates a detailed diagnostic approach, and this is usually performed by printing strips on an A4 page. An onset of paroxysmal tachycardia during physical exercise might not have been correctly identified without such a print, as it was slightly premature so the automatic diagnostic tool might have missed it. It is only when it is printed on an A4 sheet that the experienced human eye can really see the prematurity of the beat and categorise the arrhythmia correctly.

Chapter 4
Clinical Applications

The ECG Holter recording is, in the first instance, designed for *symptomatic patients* to know and correctly diagnose the arrhythmic substrate responsible of the clinical symptoms. There are two are very important factors that must be considered.

The first is that the correct diagnosis of the substrate provoking the symptomatology is only seen *a posteriori*, which means that we are not able to act clinically when the symptoms were present. Therefore, one should never use an ECG Holter as a technique to diagnose a potentially life-threatening arrhythmia. If the symptomatology is really worrying, the patient should be hospitalised in an intensive care unit for observation; the unit must also be able to treat the arrhythmia competently when it shows up.

The second factor is that the symptomatology rarely appears on a daily basis. The more frequent the symptomatology, the more opportunity there is to record it during a 24-hr ECG Holter. Therefore, it is important to enhance our chances of recording the event by taking a full and detailed history, in order to decide when the recording should be done and what type of activity the patient should engage in during the recording for the symptomatology to appear. If there is a connection between the symptomatology and the profession or sports activity, it is very important that the recording be done under relevant conditions. When recording symptomatology in a female, one must not forget to take the menstrual cycle into account because it can have a very important role in the appearance of the symptomatology.

A period of 24 hr is the minimal recording time required to get a nycthemeral profile of the basic rhythm and to be able to capture all possible triggers of arrhythmia by neurohumoral stimulation. The recorded time interval may be prolonged to 48 hr or the 24-hr recording can be repeated. It is quite often true that the presence of the recorder is seen and perceived as a nuisance by the patient, so he or she is in a neurovegetative "active" stress-related state, which may prevent the occurrence of arrhythmias. This is particularly true for the vagotonic arrhythmias, and very often the first recording does not show any arrhythmia, so one should not hesitate to repeat the recording several times. The patient is then usually much more comfortable with the device; he is relaxed and the arrhythmia can appear.

The *patient's cooperation* is indispensable because we need him to note on a logbook the activities engaged in during the day, the eventual symptomatology, and the times when medications were taken. Moreover, he should note anything

J. Adamec, R. Adamec, *ECG Holter*, DOI: 10.1007/978-0-387-78187-7_4,
© Springer Science+Business Media, LLC 2008

in connection with the recording itself. Even though the technician who places the Holter device on the patient tries to explain all this, very often in real life the patient does not understand the whole explanation, so the first logbook may be incomplete and insufficient. The doctor who forwarded the indications for the Holter recording should see the patient clinically with the Holter record to discuss his daily activities in order to interpret the arrhythmia correctly and to decide if the recording was good enough or if the procedure should be repeated.

The result of the Holter recording may be *affirmative*, which means that the recording shows a clinical symptomatology and we are able to identify an arrhythmia provoking the symptoms. Unfortunately, this happens quite rarely. On the other hand, the recording may be *exclusive*, which means that the symptomatology described adequately by the patient in the logbook has no arrhythmic substrate on the electrocardiographic tracing. This is also rare. In the majority of cases we find a *presumptuous result*, which means that during the recording the patient did not feel any specific symptomatology, but we find an arrhythmia on the tracing that could occur in its worse form and may explain the patient's symptomatology in his daily life.

It is of crucial importance in the evaluation that the tracing results are correlated with the clinical context. An ECG Holter recording during which the patient does not present any symptomatology and where we see no arrhythmia, is considered a *nil* recording and has no diagnostic value.

Patients' most frequent complaints are palpitations, and we must not forget that palpitations do not necessarily mean arrhythmias; they may be due to a sinus frequency slightly accelerated with a hypercontractibility syndrome.

A Holter recording of an asymptomatic patient, or rather a patient without symptomatology that can suggest arrhythmia, is done in situations where the discovery of cardiopathy or a specific disease is known to provoke potentially dangerous arrhythmias, even though they are asymptomatic.

When potentially serious arrhythmias are suspected, a rhythmical stress test should be considered because if the arrhythmia occurs one is at the patient's side and the treatment can be immediate. The rhythmic stress test is different from a classical stress test because the 12-lead recording must be continuous to be sure to capture the arrhythmia. The goal is to get to the maximal heart rate, so the different levels of load enhancement should be modified. We prefer to stay at a low threshold longer rather than stop the test prematurely because the patient cannot continue.

Recordings are often done on healthy individuals for various studies. Usually the subjects are athletes competing in different races. In this case, the placing of the electrodes is particularly important, as is the fixing and adapting of the recorder on the athlete's body. We have had good experience with kangaroo-type pockets on T-shirts, as, for instance, during many alpine events in the "glacier patrols race" from Zermatt to Verbier.

Chapter 5
Other ECG Recording Systems

Only rarely does the 24- or 48-hr Holter recording give the correct diagnosis in a single run, so the industry has invented recorders that can remain active for several days, up to a week. Thus, the chances of capturing the arrhythmia during the patient's symptomatology are much greater.

These devices may record different type of arrhythmias depending on their programming by reading the patient's rhythm in real time. They can also make a limited recording in time, depending on the programme for the patient's trigger, where usually the patient activates the recording device by pressing a button. The recording is continuous, so there is a memory of the recording stored in the device and its length can be programmed. When the patient presses the button, we have in memory not only this exact moment but also an interval before the onset of the trigger. This is very important because the patient often triggers the device quite late, and, as we all know, the instant of onset is the most favourable moment to correctly diagnose an arrhythmia.

It is usually useful to record an example sequence just after the device is installed on the patient and to do so in different positions, standing up, lying down, or walking around, to have a reference ECG. The patient's triggered ECG can then be compared to the basic ECG to see if there are any differences.

So that the device can stay connected to the patient for the longest possible time, there is a simple switch to turn it on and off, and the patient is instructed to do this on his or her own. The patient is also told how to change the electrodes. Nevertheless, in all cases before considering this long-duration recording *R-test*, we always recommend performing a 24-hr classical Holter because that test provides more information in a 24-hr period than the R-test. All this information is useful to correctly analyse the patient's status.

In the recent years, a new device, smaller than a pacemaker, has been developed which can be implanted and enable monitoring of the patient's rhythm for months (e.g., the Reveal system by Medtronic). The device can be interrogated at any time through telemetry, even during implantation. Unfortunately, in the clinical world it happens that we have to employ the device for an extended period, and it is only by having it continuously present under the patient's skin that we are able to arrive at the correct rhythmic diagnosis. A simple Holter recording would have been useless.

J. Adamec, R. Adamec, *ECG Holter*, DOI: 10.1007/978-0-387-78187-7_5,
© Springer Science+Business Media, LLC 2008

Chapter 6
ECG Holter and Implanted Cardioverter Defibrillators

Before performing a Holter recording on a patient with a defibrillator, it is very important to check with the device manufacturer to be sure that the recorder cannot be damaged by the defibrillator shock. This is essentially valid with the new recorders with solid statememory. Fortunately, most of the defibrillators of the latest generation have a mini-Holter system in the device. Therefore, it is often possible to get an electrocardiographic tracing just before and just after the shock. This is not a surface recording but an electric potential recording in the ventricular cavity and eventually in the atrial cavity (only with DDD PM devices).

Nevertheless, there may be an indication for a 24-hr Holter recording, especially if complicated supraventricular arrhythmias are suspected. To correctly interpret the recording one has to know the precise programming of the defibrillator device, especially the information on the stimulation program. This stimulation may be single, in doublets, or in bursts, and these programmes are there to overdrive the arrhythmias before they trigger the shock.

This correct programming of the device and its exact information must be known to the interpreter of such a Holter tracing. The information must always be correlated with the mini-Holter memory of the device, and only then can the arrhythmic problem be addressed correctly.

J. Adamec, R. Adamec, *ECG Holter*, DOI: 10.1007/978-0-387-78187-7_6,
© Springer Science+Business Media, LLC 2008

Chapter 7
ECG Report Example

Even though the automatic system gives more and more information, it is a fundamental requirement that the cardiologist responsible for the interpretation of a Holter examination verify all the facts elicited by the automatic reader and correct the report to make it complete.

Basic Rhythm

- Sinus rhythm, atrial fibrillation, or other
- Identical rhythm during all recording or rhythm alternation in time
- Alternation particularity (day, night, during bradycardia or tachycardia)
- Nycthemeral profile: its aspect and particularities
- Cardiac frequency: maximal and minimal heart rate in correlation with the physical activities of the patient
- Extrasystolies: as the human interpreter, one must either accept or reject the automatic interpretation, for both ventricular and supraventricular extrasystolies

Supraventricular Extrasystolies

- State the number in words

  - Sporadic
  - Rare (1–4 extrasystolies/hr)
  - Frequent (4–40 extrasystolies/hr)
  - Numerous (40–140 extrasystolies/hr)
  - Very numerous (more than 400 extrasystolies/hr)

- State the connections

  - Isolated
  - In doublets
  - Interpolated
  - Bi-, tri-, quadrigeminism
  - Blocked

J. Adamec, R. Adamec, *ECG Holter*, DOI: 10.1007/978-0-387-78187-7_7,
© Springer Science+Business Media, LLC 2008

- State the origin

  - Atrial
  - Junctional
  - With intraventricular aberration

Ventricular Extrasystolies

- State the number in words

  - Sporadic
  - Rare (1–4 extrasystolies/hr)
  - Frequent (4–40 extrasystolies/hr)
  - Numerous (40–140 extrasystolies/hr)
  - Very numerous (more than 400 extrasystolies/hr)

- State the connections

  - Isolated
  - In doublets
  - Interpolated
  - Bi-, tri-, quadrigeminism

- Morphology

  - Monomorphic
  - Bi-, polymorphic

Tachycardias

The cardiologist must either accept or correct the automatic reading and especially correctly state the origin of the tachycardias (supraventricular tachycardias vs. ventricular tachycardias).

Supraventricular Tachycardias

- Number of episodes
- Duration of episodes
- Tachycardia heart rate frequency
- Presence or absence of sinus rhythm just after the stopping of the tachycardia and how long does it stay (state its length of time in seconds)
- Onset particularities
- Substrate

  - Atrial
  - Atrial block
  - Dual pathway

     ○ Preexcitation syndrome as for instance WPW
     ○ Presence of aberration
     ○ Unknown

Ventricular Tachycardias

- Number of episodes
- Episode duration

     ○ Sustained vs. nonsustained

- Tachycardia heart rate frequency

     ○ Onset particularities

- Morphology r/t, r/p

Pauses

- Duration in milliseconds
- Origin
- Number of pauses

Blocks

- Level of the block, either sinoatrial or atrioventricular
- Degree and type
- Particularity
- Bundle branch (phase 3 or 4)

Preexcitation: Present vs. Absent

ST Segment

- Appreciation
- Specificity for the ischemia
- Number of episodes
- Episode duration

Symptomatology

- Noted by patient on the logbook
- Is there an ECG substrate at the moment of the symptomatology?

Patient's Physical Activity

- Consequence on the heart rate frequency

Technical Appreciation of the Recording Quality

General Comments

Chapter 8
Conclusion

As the full medical history in a clinical examination is a crucially important factor at the patient's bedside, we hope that we have convinced our readers of the cardinal role of electrocardiographic diagnoses in clinical rhythmology.

Nowadays, in the medical field as in real life, we have a tendency to be overwhelmed by a continuous flow of information, and it is essential that we distinguish the real messages from the parasites.

What looks scintillating and seductive on an automatic reading must not make us forget the basic principles of a correct interpretation.

J. Adamec, R. Adamec, *ECG Holter*, DOI: 10.1007/978-0-387-78187-7_8,
© Springer Science+Business Media, LLC 2008

Bibliography

1. Holter NJ: New method for heart studies. *Science*, 1961; **134**: 1214–1229.
2. Bleifer SB, Bleifer DJ, Hansmann DR, Sheppard JJ, and Karpmann HL: Diagnosis of occult arrhythmias by Holter electrocardiography. *Prog Cardiovasc Dis* 1974; **16**: 569–599.
3. Lipski J, Cohen L, Espinoso J, Motro M, Dack S, and Donoso E: Value of Holter monitoring in assessing cardiac arrhythmias in symptomatic patients. *Am J Cardiol* 1976; **37**: 102–109.
4. Winkle RA: Antiarrhythmic drug effect mimicked by spontaneous variability of ventricular ectopy. *Circulation* 1978; **57**: 1116–1121.
5. Oter R and Telleria R: Contribution of Holter's system of Sinus sinus node disease, **In**: Bayes A and Cosin NJ Eds: *Diagnosis and Treatment of Cardiac Arrhythmias*. Pergamon Press, Oxford, 1980.
6. Leclercq JF and Coumel Ph: L'enregistrement Holter en rythmologie. *Laboratoires Labaz*, Paris, 1980.
7. Adamec R: L'enregistrement èlectrocardiographique continu (système de Holter) dans le diagnostic de l'origine des malaises et des syncopes. *Med & Hyg* 1981; **39**: 4074–4078.
8. Wenger NK, Mock MB, and Ring-Ouist I: *Ambulatory Electrocardiographic Recording*. Year Book Medical Publishers, Chicago, 1981.
9. Fillette F, Fontaine G, and Tardieu B: *L'essentiel sur l'enregistrement Holter de l'ECG*. Masson, Paris, 1983.
10. Sheffield LT, Berson A, Bragg-Remschel D, Gillette PC, et al.: Recommendation for standards of instrumentation and practice in the use of ambulatory electrocardiography. *Circulation* 1985; **71**: 626A–636A.
11. Hilgard J, Ezrim D, and Denes P: Significance of ventricular pauses of three seconds or more detected on twenty-four-hour Holter recordings. *Am J Cardiol* 1985 **55**: 1005–1008.
12. Houille F, Louvet JM, and Ducardonnet A: L'enregistrement Holter normal et pathologique. *Biosedra Cardiologie*, Malakoff, 1986.
13. Guidelines for Ambulatory Electrocardiography: A Report of the American College of Cardiology/American Heart Association Task Force on Assessment of Diagnostic and Therapeutic Cardiovascular Procedures (Subcommittee on Ambulatory Electrocardiography). *J Am Coll Cardiol* 1989; **13**: 249–258.
14. Leclercq JF and Coumel Ph: Ambulatory electrocardiogram monitoring. **In**: MacFarlane PW and Veitsch Lanrie Eds: *Comprehensive Electrocardiology: Theory and Practice in Health and Disease*. Pergamon Press, New York, 1989.
15. MacFarlane PN: Lead systems. **In**: MacFarlane PW and Veitsch Lanrie Eds: *Comprehensive Electrocardiology: Theory and Practice in Health and Disease*. Pergamon Press, New York, 1989.
16. Ward DE: Ambulatory monitoring of the electrocardiogram **In**: Julian DG, Camm AJ, Fox KM, Hall RJ, and Poole-Nilson Ph Eds: *Diseases of the Heart*. Bailliere-Tindall, London, 1989.

17. Coumel Ph: Role of the autonomic nervous system in paroxysmal atrial fibrillation, **In**: Touboul P and Waldo AL Eds: *Atrial Arrhythmias: Current Concepts and Management.* Mosby CV, St Louis, 1990.

18. Coumel Ph: Electrocardiographie et informatique, **In**: Denolin H, Coumel Ph, Bourdarias JP, and Lenaers A Eds: *Methodes d'investigation en cardiologie.* Maloine, Paris, 1993.

19. Quiret JC and Bemasconi P: L'enregistrement électrocardiographique par la méthode de Holter dans l'insuffisance coronarienne, **In**: Denolin H, Coumel Ph, Bourdarias JP, and Lenaers A Eds: *Méthodes d'investigation en cardiologie.* Maloine, Paris, 1993.

20. Medvedovsky JL and Leclercq JF: L'ECG de longue durée:arythmies et leur évaluation quantitative, **In**: Denolin H, Coumel Ph, Bourdarias JP, and Lenaers A Eds: *Méthuds d'investigation en cardiologie.* Maloine, Paris, 1993.

21. Morillo CA, Klein GJ, Thakur RK, Li H, Zardini M, and Yeer R: Mechanism of "inappropriate" sinus tachycardia: role of sympathovagal balance. *Circulation* 1994; **17**: 1569–1576.

22. Association for the Advancement of Medical Instrumentation. American National Standard: Ambulatory Electrocardiographs. Arlington, VA, ANSI/AAMI, EC38, 1994.

23. Prystowsky EN: *The Role of Event Recording in the Diagnosis and Management of Transient Arrhythmias.* Communications Media for Education, New Jersey, 1994.

24. Barold SS: Evaluation of Pacemaker Function by Holter Recordings, **In**: Moss AJ and Stern Sh Eds: *Non invasive Electrocardiology.* Saunders, London, 1996.

25. Deedwania PC: Ischemia detected by Holter monitoring in coronary artery disease, **In**: Moss AJ and Stern S Eds. *Noninvasive Electrocardiology.* Saunders, London, 1996.

26. Noble RJ and Zipes DP: Long-Term continuous electrocardiographic recording, **In**: Schlant RC and Alexander RW Eds. *The Heart,* Mc-Graw-Hill, New York, 1994.

27. Kennedy HL: Holter recorders and analytic systems, **In**: Moss AJ and Stern S Eds: *Noninvasive Electrocardiology.* Saunders, London, 1996.

28. Te-Chuan Chou: Ambulatory electrocardiography, **In**: Te-Chuan Chou Ed: *Electrocardiography in Clinical Practice.* Saunders, Philadelphia, 1996.

29. Badilini F, Zareba W, Titlebaum EL, and Moss AJ: Analysis of ST segment variability in Holter recordings, **In**: Moss AJ and Stern S Eds: *Noninvasive Electrocardiology.* Saunders, London, 1996.

30. Moss AJ: Clinical utility of ST segment monitoring, **In**: Moss AJ and Stern S Eds: *Noninvasive Electrocardiology.* Saunders, London, 1996.

31. Mulcahy D and Ouyyumi AA: Clinical implications of circadian rhythms detected by ambulatory monitoring techniques, **In**: Moss AJ and Stern S Eds: *Noninvasive Electrocardiology.* Saunders, London, 1996.

32. Bayes De Luna: Holter electrocardiography and other related techniques, **In**: Bayes De Luna Ed: *Clinical Electrocardiography: A Textbook.* Futura, Armonk, 1998.

33. Noble RJ and Zipes DP: Long-term continuous electrocardiographic recording, **In**: Alexander RW, Schlant RC, and Fuser V Eds: *Hurst's The Heart.* Mc Graw-Hill, NY, 1998.

34. ACC/AHA Guidelines for ambulatory electrocardiography. *J Am Coll Cardio,* 1999: **34**: 912–948.

Index

With thanks to Tess who supervised the English language translation

Printed in the United States